To the memory of Edward Mapother and Frederick Mott

Madness
to Mental Illness

A history of the Royal College of Psychiatrists

Thomas Bewley

RCPsych Publications

© The Royal College of Psychiatrists 2008

RCPsych Publications is an imprint of the Royal College of Psychiatrists,
17 Belgrave Square, London SW1X 8PG
http://www.rcpsych.ac.uk

British Library Cataloguing-in-Publication Data.
A catalogue record for this book is available from the British Library.
ISBN 978-1-904671-35-0

Distributed in North America by Balogh International Inc.

The views presented in this book do not necessarily reflect those of the Royal College of
Psychiatrists, and the publishers are not responsible for any error of omission or fact.

The Royal College of Psychiatrists is a charity registered in England and Wales (228636) and in
Scotland (SC038369).

Printed by in the UK by Cromwell Press Ltd, Trowbriedge, Wiltshire.

Contents

Tables, boxes, plates and online archives

Online archives

People

1. William Tuke (1732–1822)
2. Robert Gardiner Hill (1811–1878)
3. John Conolly (1794-1866) (non-restraint)
4. Samuel Hitch (1800-1881) (founder of the Association)
5. Shaftesbury, (1801-1885) (Anthony Ashley-Cooper, Seventh earl of Shaftesbury, with his diary on his 50th birthday)
6. John Bucknill (1817-1897) (first editor of the Journal)
7. Daniel Hack Tuke (1817–1895)
8. Sir James Crichton-Browne (1840–1938) (The Wakefield Triangle)
9. Thomas Smith Clouston (1840–1915)
10. Conolly Norman (1852–1908)
11. Henry Maudsley (1835–1918)
12. Frederick Mott (1853–1926)
13. Edward Mapother (1881–1940)
14. Aubrey Lewis (1900–1975)
15. Alexander Walk (1901–1982)
16. Martin Roth (1917–2006)

Important legal cases of the 19th century

17. James Hadfield
18. Edward Oxford (law and insanity)
19. Daniel McNaughten (The McNaughten Rules)

Asylum practice

20. Patients' views
21. Kilkenny and Ballinasloe district asylums
22. The penultimate medical superintendent (Dr J. E. S. Lloyd, 1901–1971)
23. Asylum dance
24. Asylum rules
    a. Cardiff 1919
    b. London 1966
25. Association and College committees/structures
    a. Divisions
    b. Specialties
        i.   Standing committees and sections
        ii. Forensic

Foreword

Sheila Hollins

Dr Thomas Bewley has written an account of psychiatry in Britain which covers the past two hundred years and investigates the many changes from asylum care to the psychiatry practised today. He has taken a wide view of all aspects of the profession and sees value in an integrated psychological and biological approach to treating people with mental illnesses. He has concentrated on the major organisations responsible for the care of people with mental disorders and has shown how different branches of the profession (learning disability psychiatry, child psychiatry, psychotherapy, forensic psychiatry and addictions psychiatry) have developed. Academic developments in teaching and research are also covered. Other changes mentioned in the book include the relationship that psychiatrists have with patients or service users and those caring for them, both their families and those in other professions.

Although this book has been written for psychiatrists there is much in it that should be of interest to all those who are involved in any way with people with mental ill health. Earlier theories about mental illnesses are covered, as well as the treatments that, partly because of the development of scientific methods of evaluation of therapies, have been abandoned. For example we know now that some treatments work for a limited number of people, but there are also placebo effects; it is essential to know which are most effective.

The moral from this book is that society must care better for all those disadvantaged by mental disorders, as well as endeavouring to find new and better methods of treatment. Dr Bewley surmises that these will be likely to include social care, access to work, occupational and other therapies as well as advances in medical and psychological treatments. All those concerned with and about people with mental illness could learn something from this fascinating exploration of the history of psychiatry.

Preface

Some books are to be tasted, others to be swallowed, and some few to be chewed and digested.

Francis Bacon

When I was invited in 1996 to write an account of the College's history there was no official history of it or its forerunners. There was much information in the College archives and in its journal (the *British Journal of Psychiatry*, previously the *Journal of Mental Science*). I intended to write a short book, mainly of interest to College members, which I hoped might also be useful for a wider readership. It provides an account of the changes in psychiatric practice in the UK over 200 years with the development of an association which became a Royal College. I have brought together the quintessence of the changes (warts and all) with the history of the organisation most involved with the mentally ill. The College's charter notes that its objects and purposes are to 'advance the science and practice of psychiatry, further public education therein and promote study and research work in psychiatry.' This book could, therefore, further public education.

There are many people who might have some interest in such an account: patients and their families, friends and carers; and others concerned about mental health issues, for example physicians, general practitioners, community nurses, psychologists, psychoanalysts, probation officers, lawyers and the police. All of these should have some interest in a history of the care, and at times control, of the mentally ill.

I started by drafting a full account of everything that might be relevant, which meant I had too much information for a short book. I consigned much of this material to appendices (online archives) available on the College website (www.rcpsych.ac.uk/historyarchives).

At the end of some chapters I note articles and books that I have very much relied upon and would recommend for further reading. I hope this will encourage the readers to extract as much, or as little, as they need, whether they decide to taste, swallow or chew and digest. The online archives include accounts written by other authors and addressing issues covered in the book, but in greater detail, with references to sources where further information is available.

T. B.

Acknowledgements

A novice copies but a master craftsman steals.

Michaelangelo

There is little original in this book and I have relied heavily on various sources. I found much valuable information in the two volumes of the *150 Years of British Psychiatry* (eds G. Berrios & H. Freeman). The late Alexander Walk had trawled the College archives for articles about the Medico–Psychological Association in the 19th century and I used his material to research this book. I have relied very heavily on Trevor Turner, E. H. Renvoise, William Parry Jones and Henry Rollin, and I am heavily indebted to all of them.

Those providing me with further specialised information about the College and its forerunners included Fiona Subotsky, who helped me shorten and edit what I had drafted and also wrote an account of College finances. Margaret Harcourt Williams dredged the archives for me and also wrote an account of the College premises. Other appendices about the College divisions and specialties were provided by many people. For example, Allan Tait had written an excellent account of the Scottish Division which I shamelessly plundered to use as an example of divisional activities.

I was much helped by those who looked at and improved drafts of individual chapters and appendices. These included David Goldberg, Alan Beveridge, John Gunn, John Wing, Peter Rohde, Peter Noble, Dinesh Bhugra, Richard Williams, Robert Bluglass, Michael Crowe, Stirling Moorey, Frank Margison, Anton Obholzer, Eammon Fottrell, Tom Arie, Brice Pitt, Fiona Subotsky, Tony Cox, Lionel Hersov, Ilana Crome, Hamid Ghodse, Andrew Johns, Joan Bicknell, Alan Heaton Ward, Ben Sacks, Yvonne Wiley, David Tait, Marcus Webb and Chris Freeman.

Among those who provided drafts for the faculties and sections were Robert Bluglass, Michael Crowe, Ilana Crome, Peter Snowden, Mary Lindsey, Peter Carpenter, Alan Heaton Ward, Dinesh Bhugra, Caroline Lindsey, Andrew Fairbairn, Laurence Measey, Alan Howe, Sheila Davies, Howard Ring, David Veale, Jonathan Pedder, Malcolm Pines, Mike Farrell, Tom Arie, David Jolley, Stephen Kingsbury, Susan Benbow, Geoffrey Lloyd, Eilish Gilvarry, Tom Carnwath and Yvonne Wiley. I have also received much help with the accounts of the College divisions from Philip Sugarman,

Christopher Mayer, Dermot McGovern, Miriam Silke and Philip Greenberg. I am much indebted to all of them.

Many other people helped me as well, including Lucy Hastings, Thomas Kennedy, Paul Lelliott, Gerry Low Beer, David Walk, Fiby Hare, Susan Floate, John Howells, Constance Roth, Raymond Levy, Bob Kendell, Brian Barraclough, Peggy Walk, Kingsley Jones, Morwenna Rogers, Alexandra Cohen, Laura Hulse and Emily Johns.

A first draft for the book was read by three anonymous referees as well as Stephen Lock, Henry Rollin, Jim Birley and Elizabeth Shore. Their comments were extremely helpful. Finally I would also like to thank those who supported me generously over a very long time: Vanessa Cameron, Margaret Harcourt Williams, Susie Stewart, Mary Ayres and some members of my family, including Beulah, Susan and Henry Bewley.

Introduction

They pour medicines of which they know little into patients of whom they know less to treat conditions of which they know nothing at all.

Voltaire

Two hundred years of psychiatry in Britain

In Great Britain and Ireland the history of psychiatry is bound up with the history of one organisation – the Medico-Psychological Association, which started in 1841 as an association of medical officers of asylums and hospitals. Since its inception it has reflected and influenced the way in which psychiatric disorders have been perceived and managed in the UK.

In the early 19th century, evangelicalism played a major part in English lunacy reform and in changes towards a more rational and humane legislation concerning people with mental illness. It helped to form the basis of 'moral treatment' (a psychological approach), which was a critical concept in the process of transition to the modern era. This alternative approach to insanity postulated that physicians, by their moral example, would appeal to the 'human spirit' present in patients despite madness, and the asylum regime would guide their troubled minds back to sanity. This 'moral' view was held mostly by minorities such as Quakers, Unitarians and other dissenters. Anthony Ashley-Cooper, 7th Earl of Shaftesbury, was a major figure in this movement in 19th-century Britain. He was a layman who, for the greater part of his life, was heavily involved in ensuring that the mentally ill were cared for humanely and with kindness in the hope that, after being rescued from neglect, squalor or imprisonment, they would respond to good food, clean air and education. He was a supporter of those doctors who favoured moral treatment rather than restraint.[1] The principles of the moral treatment were noble, but sociologists argue that actual practice could be morally inadequate and characterised by cruelty and neglect.[2] Their view was that the humanitarianism of the asylum, the effectiveness of psychological medicine and the validity of 'community care' as a non-institutional treatment alternative were myths. Psychiatrists were in it to look after themselves.

---

1   Online archive 5. Shaftesbury.
2   Scull, A. (1993) *The Most Solitary of Afflictions*. Yale University Press.

In documenting the history of the College, original accounts of events are included where possible. Thus nearly two centuries of activity are covered, with accounts of major changes in the work of psychiatrists and in the institutions involved. Doctors often failed to understand the mentally ill. Voltaire's cynical view of medicine applies equally to all branches and specialties, but psychiatrists were regarded as no better, and sometimes worse than other doctors. The 'warts and all' view of the profession adopted in this book includes some useless treatments, foolish views and other shortcomings. However, there have been improvements, though not always as significant as may have been hoped for. It would not be possible to chart the transition of the Association into the College without at the same time explaining changes in the practice of psychiatry. Therefore, where relevant, most chapters contain a short account of the state of the mentally ill at a given period, and how they were dealt with by society as a whole and by the medical profession. This includes the remedies and the methods of care or of detention available at the time and also some of the theories and hypothetical models of treatment.

The Association of Medical Officers of Asylums and Hospitals for the Insane was established in 1841, but the building of public asylums had started a century earlier. During the 19th century there was a marked increase in the numbers of asylums and patients admitted. Previously, those with severe mental illness who could not be looked after by their families were either admitted to private mental hospitals or were contained in prisons or workhouses. An important role of the early asylum movement was to transfer the mentally ill from prisons and madhouses to mental hospitals, and in the earliest days of the Association, there was great optimism that treating patients early and humanely would enable them to recover. The membership of the Association was initially restricted to medical officers who worked in asylums. They intended to meet once a year, but in the early years meetings were not always held regularly. A major change followed the Association's decision to produce its own journal in 1853. This was followed by changing the name in 1865 to the Medico-Psychological Association (MPA), a title it retained for the next 60 years, until in 1926 it acquired the royal charter and became the Royal Medico-Psychological Association (RMPA). There were no changes in its functioning till 1971, when a new charter was granted thus establishing the Royal College of Psychiatrists.

Since 1841, there have been major advancements in the methods of treatment available to the mentally ill. By the late 19th century the initial optimism that the ability to treat patients early in new asylums would lead to better outcomes had changed gradually to a realisation that some people were not responsive to any treatment and that there was a growing number of patients with severe long-term illnesses who required continuing care. For half a century a pessimistic view of what could be achieved prevailed and there was a tendency to see asylums as repositories for chronically ill patients. Before the Second World War there were few specific treatments. One major advancement occurred in the treatment of cerebral syphilis (General

Paralysis of the Insane, GPI) – this devastating and fatal illness responded to malarial treatment. Furthermore, electroconvulsive therapy (ECT) was introduced just before the Second World War and in the 1950s a range of new drugs became available. Antidepressants and other antipsychotic drugs, which could modify some of the symptoms of schizophrenia and other major illnesses, were developed. Some treatments came in vogue for a time but were subsequently discarded. The idea that mental illness was caused by bacterial infections ('focal sepsis') was one such; insulin coma therapy for schizophrenia was another. Psychosurgery, crude and uncertain operations, was also a form of treatment and was used indiscriminately in the 1940s and 1950s in people with severe mental illness.

In the 20th century there were significant changes in psychiatry. The first was the development in England of a more scientific approach to the subject, exemplified by the establishment of the Maudsley Hospital and the Institute of Psychiatry. The endeavours of Henry Maudsley, Frederick Mott, Edward Mapother and Aubrey Lewis led to a core of better trained psychiatrists, with knowledgeable junior members of the profession who were instrumental in the change from a tired Association to an active College. Evidence-based medicine, particularly the development of the randomised controlled trial, has led in psychiatry, as in all other branches of medicine, to a better understanding of treatments and allowed us to see which are the most effective. Another major change worldwide has been a move away from asylums to the siting of psychiatric units in general hospitals, with hostels for the chronically ill in the community. Some problems remain the same today as they were two hundred years ago; the most intractable is the continuing care of those who do not get better. There has always been a tendency to underestimate the difficulties of looking after those most severely and chronically ill.

Further reading

Scull, A. (1993) *The Most Solitary of Afflictions*. Yale University Press.

CHAPTER 1

Historical background
1780–1840

In the 18th and early 19th centuries, people with mental illness could be cast out from society. If harmless, they were ignored and left to cope as best they could; if considered dangerous, they were confined, sometimes in degrading conditions. Confinement was a way of removing them from society; treatment was rudimentary and mechanical restraint was sometimes necessary. The mental illness of King George III helped to focus public and political attention on the problems of the mentally ill – politicians and doctors began to be more active and asylums were built. This led to the foundation in 1841 of the Association of Medical Officers of Asylums and Hospitals for the Insane.

Previous provision

Private madhouses had been a feature of British life for several centuries and they became increasingly common during the 18th century. Such establishments catered both for the affluent and for paupers if boarded out by their parishes who paid their fees. This 'trade in lunacy' was run for profit by lay people such as clergymen, as well as by doctors, and the institutions ranged in size from one to over a hundred patients. Accommodation could be sparse and unsuitable for the purpose and patients might be subjected to harsh treatment and mechanical restraint.

Although the Hospital of St Mary of Bethlem (Bedlam) in London had cared for the mentally ill since at least 1403, it was not until the 18th century that hospital facilities for the insane began to be seriously provided, and even this was on a relatively small scale. Hospital institutions were founded in Norwich in 1713; at St Luke's in London in 1751; Manchester in 1766; Newcastle in 1767; York in 1777; and Liverpool in 1790. Until around 1812, there was not a single public county or borough asylum for the insane in England, though there were several hospitals for the mentally afflicted founded by royal or private benevolence – for example, the Royal Hospitals of Bridewell and Bethlem, St Luke's Hospital in London, the Quaker foundations of the Retreat and Bootham in York, and the Bethel Hospital in Norwich. However, institutional care of the mentally ill in such asylums or private madhouses was the exception rather than the rule. The majority of the mentally ill and those with learning disability (called 'idiots', 'imbeciles' or 'feeble minded') were looked after by their families or were confined in workhouses, poorhouses and prisons.

Unease about the state in which many lunatics were kept led to the 1774 Act of Parliament, under which five commissioners from the Royal College of Physicians inspected private madhouses in London, and justices visited and licensed those in the provinces. Though not successful in eliminating abuses, this Act was a forerunner for the later system of inspection of asylums.

In the early 19th century, a major factor in bringing mental illness to public attention was the illness of George III, a popular monarch who suffered recurrent periods of mania (now considered probably to be caused by porphyria) that his physicians were unable to control. They sought the advice of the Reverend Doctor Francis Willis, who ran an asylum in Lincolnshire. He is said to have told the king that he was in urgent need of medical treatment because his ideas were deranged and that he must control himself or be put in a straitjacket. The prominence of the king's illness and its treatment focused attention on the problem and led to questioning about the lunacy laws.

The Retreat and non-restraint

In Britain, the founding of the Retreat at York in 1796 by William Tuke, a Quaker and a layman, with the development there of 'moral treatment', showed that asylum patients could be cared for more humanely. When Tuke's grandson Samuel published details of the institution and its methods in *Description of the Retreat* in 1813, the concepts of moral treatment reached a wider audience. Despite its small size and other atypical characteristics, the Retreat began to act as a model which many future asylums attempted to reproduce.[1]

The views of the original promoters of this establishment shed some light on the psychological, moral and medical treatment available to the mentally ill at that time. Although they were aware that abuses existed in many asylums, they expected that there would be people from whose practice they might learn and by whose instructions they might be guided in the main principles of their moral and medical treatment. The system at that time generally adopted relied on the principle of fear to govern the insane. The practical consequence deduced from this was that attendants should initially relate to patients with an appearance of austerity and perhaps the display of personal strength; in some cases of violent excitement, force would be the most suitable method of control. At the beginning the Retreat assented to the general correctness of these views and although they were modified by the good sense and feeling of the management committee, they were acted upon to an extent that we can hardly contemplate without surprise today.

The second superintendent, or chief nurse, at the Retreat was George Jepson. Before his appointment to the Retreat in 1797 he had doubts as to whether this severe system of management was necessary. He had observed

---

1   Online archive 1. William Tuke.

that wild animals were most easily tamed by gentle methods and judging by analogy, he inferred that a man without reason might be influenced by the same means. He adopted a system that presumed the patient to be generally capable to be influenced through the kindly affections of the heart and also in a considerable degree through the medium of the understanding. His approach to the treatment of patients was a mixture of moral, educational and behavioural methods – an early example of a psychological approach. The success of the Retreat convinced many that institutional care was the ideal method of treatment for the mentally ill.

Legislation, regulation and public provision

The first reference to lunatics can be found in a statute of Edward II (1320) when it was enacted that the property and estates of lunatics were vested in the Crown. There was no lunacy legislation proper till 1744 when a bill for 'regulating madhouses' was passed to regulate private asylums in which abuses were prevalent. The Act was not effective since anyone could get a licence to open an asylum. The Royal College of Physicians of London received reports of abuses but could do little. This Act also authorised any two justices to apprehend pauper lunatics who could be detained. The purpose of this Act was the protection of society, as it provided for those who 'are so far disordered in their senses that they may be too dangerous to be permitted to go abroad'. There was then no further legislation until 1808 when a bill, usually referred to as Wynn's Act, 'for the better care and maintenance of lunatics being paupers or criminals in England' was passed. The opening preamble read:

'Whereas the practice of confining such Lunatics and other insane persons as are chargeable to their respective parishes in Gaols, Houses of Correction, Poor-houses, and Houses of Industry, is highly dangerous and inconvenient, and whereas it is expedient that provision should be made for the care and maintenance of such persons, and for the erecting of proper houses for their reception … it shall be lawful for the Justices, assembled in Quarter Sessions of the County, to take into consideration the expediency of providing a Lunatic Asylum in such County.'

Under this Act, magistrates were allowed to build a rate-supported asylum in each county to cope with the large number of pauper lunatics. As the Act was discretionary, only nine English counties complied, but concern for the plight of the mentally ill was increasing. The first county asylum was opened in 1812 in Nottinghamshire and by 1841 a further 13 had been added (Box 1.1).

A Parliamentary Select Committee of Inquiry, held between 1815 and 1816, found further evidence of abuses, not only in private madhouses and workhouses but also at the Bethlem Hospital and the York Asylum. The result of the investigation into the latter led to all officers there being dismissed and attention being focused on the use of bars, chains and handcuffs and

Box 1.1 Public asylums opened between 1812 and 1841

1812	Nottingham County (Sneiton)
1814	Norfolk County
1816	Lancaster County
1818	Stafford County
1818	York, County (Wakefield)
1820	Cornwall County
1823	Lincoln County
1823	Gloucester County
1829	Chester County
1829	Suffolk County
1830	Middlesex County (Hanwell)
1832	Dorset County
1833	Kent County (Barming Heath)
1841	Surrey County (Wandsworth)

on the filth, nakedness and misery inflicted on the inmates. This convinced many of the need for greater state intervention in the care of the mentally ill, and also for an improved system of inspection of institutions by a national body. Opposition from various quarters defeated attempts to pass legislation and it was not until 1828 that the new Commission in Lunacy was able to license and supervise private madhouses in the metropolitan area, although the Act did not apply to county asylums. This omission was remedied in the Lunacy Acts in 1845 (Lunacy Act and Irish Lunatics Asylums Act), and the County Asylums Act in the same year made the building of county and borough asylums for pauper lunatics compulsory.

Doctors and treatment

Towards the latter part of the 18th century, some members of the medical profession were also beginning to show interest in the diagnostic, clinical, therapeutic, and legal aspects of the care of the insane. There was a growth in medically-run asylums, a development in medical literature on the subject, and medico-legal involvement in court cases. The recognition that the mind is a function of the brain enhanced this process, so that it became increasingly accepted by doctors, and to a lesser extent by the public, that mental illness was in fact a disease and thus fell within the province of the medical profession. Doctors were given an important inspection and supervisory role in relation to metropolitan private madhouses under the 1828 Act, and then under the Lunacy Act 1845. This made it mandatory that each county asylum should have a resident medical officer and gave official recognition to the dominant position of the medical profession in the diagnosis and treatment of mental illness. Doctors (physician superintendents) were in charge and were expected to live on the premises. This group was the force behind the establishment of the Association of Medical Officers of Asylums and Hospitals for the Insane in 1841.

Mechanical restraint was widely used at the time. Some inmates were chained to stone floors, to the walls of their cells, to the bars of a cage, or to heavy wooden trough bedsteads. This was not always restricted to periods of maniacal excitement but could continue for years, sometimes for life. The comparative efficacy of chains, handcuffs, iron girdles, collars and strait-waistcoats was discussed. Some of the public asylums followed the example of Tuke at the Retreat and endeavoured to treat patients without recourse to restraint. For many years, arguments between the proponents and opponents of the movement appeared in the pages of the *Journal of Mental Science*. Dr Gardiner Hill, the superintendent of the asylum at Lincoln, was the first to organise his hospital in such a way that no restraint was used. He was followed by the probably better known John Conolly, who at a larger asylum (Hanwell, with 2000 beds) was able in the course of 13 years (six as a medical superintendent and seven as a visiting physician) to do away with all forms of restraint.[2]

Drug and other treatments

There was little in the way of drug treatment. Sedative drugs such as laudanum (tincture of opium) could only be given orally and overactive, overexcited and deluded patients were unlikely to take them. In the early 19th century some drugs could be administered to willing patients for their supposed calming or stimulating properties but these would only have a temporary effect. It was only after the development of the hypodermic syringe that it was possible to give patients a drug without their consent.

Baths in various forms were widely used in asylums, mainly to calm excitement. One of these was the 'bath of surprise', a reservoir of water into which the patient was suddenly precipitated while standing on its moveable and treacherous cover. There were also other various types of baths – the plunge bath, the shower bath and the douche (a jet or stream of water applied to some part of the body generally for medicinal purposes), all with water temperatures below 75°F, and the hot bath, the warm bath and the tepid bath with temperatures at or above 85°F. At that time there was no remedy of more universal employment in the treatment of the insane than

---

2   Online archive 2. Robert Gardiner Hill & 3. John Conolly.

the shower bath. It could be seen fixed in every ward of an Engl
asylum and was used in nearly every form of illness.

The late 18th and early 19th centuries saw the beginnings of a
more humane approach to mental illness and it was against this backgro__
of increasing legislation and asylum building that moves began to form a
body to represent those in charge of the running of asylums and hospitals
for the insane.

Further reading

Hodder, E. (1887) *The Life and Work of the 7th Earl of Shaftesbury.* 3 vols. Cornell.

MacAlpine, I. & Hunter, R. (1969) *George III and the Mad Business.* Penguin Press.

Parry-Jones, W. (1972) *The Trade in Lunacy. A Study of Private Madhouses in England in the Eighteenth and Nineteenth Centruries.* Routledge & Kegan Paul.

Tuke, D. H. (1855) William Tuke, the founder of the York Retreat. *Journal of Psychological Medicine and Mental Pathology,* **8**, 507–512.

Tuke, D. H. (1858) On warm and cold baths in the treatment of insanity. *Journal of Mental Science,* **5**, 102–114.

Walk, A. (1961) The history of mental nursing. *Journal of Mental Science,* **446**, 1–17.

Walk, A. & Walker, D. L. (1961) Gloucester and the beginnings of the RMPA. *Journal of Mental Science,* **449**, 603–632.

Association of Medical Officers of Asylums and Hospitals for the Insane
1841–1865

Following the increase in asylum building some doctors decided to form a body to represent medical men working in asylums and hospitals for the insane. In 1841 Dr Samuel Hitch, resident superintendent of the Gloucestershire General Lunatic Asylum proposed the setting up of an association of 'Medical Gentlemen connected with Lunatic Asylums'. Dr Hitch was an energetic and enlightened physician who was prepared to persevere in the search for better treatment, better research and more accurate statistics to improve the lot of the mentally ill. He sent a circular to 88 resident medical superintendents and visiting physicians in 44 asylums and hospitals, 26 in England, 11 in Ireland and 7 in Scotland. This circular was forwarded to each medical officer of a lunatic asylum in Britain as far as they were known and to several physicians on the continent. His letter explained his proposals.[1]

Gloucester, June 19th 1841

Dear Sir,

It having been long felt desirable that the Medical Gentlemen connected with Lunatic Asylums should be better known to each other – should communicate more freely the results of their individual experience – should cooperate in collecting statistical information relating to insanity and above all should assist each other in improving the treatment of the insane – several Gentlemen who have the conduct of Lunatic Asylums have determined on making an attempt to form "an Association of the Medical Officers of Lunatic Asylums".

For this purpose they propose to meet annually at the time and place the "British Association for the Cultivation of Science" shall select for holding their meetings and to hold a first, or preliminary Meeting this year on the 29th of July next at Devonport.

I have been requested by these Gentlemen to learn how far their brethren will cooperate with them, and I shall feel it a personal kindness therefore if you will, as soon as possible, give me your opinion upon this proposed Association, and also inform me if you will give it your support.

I beg to remain, Sir,

Your obedient and faithful servant,

Samuel Hitch, Resident Physician, Gloucestershire General Lunatic Asylum

---

1   Online archive 4. Samuel Hitch.

The Committee of the Gloucestershire Medical Asylum agreed to provide the venue for a preliminary meeting to be held in their institution on 27 July 1841 to prepare the ground for the inaugural meeting at Devonport. Forty-five of the initially approached 88 doctors were prepared to join the association, three refused and 40 did not reply. Only four of those willing to join would attend the meeting at Devonport. A preliminary meeting was, therefore, held at the Gloucester Asylum on 27 July 1841. Six doctors were present – Handwick Shute (the chair), Samuel Hitch of the Gloucester Asylum, Samuel Gaskell (Lancaster), Thomas Powell (Nottingham), John Thurnam (York Retreat) and Frederick Wintle (Oxford). As the four doctors who had agreed to go to Devonport were all present at this preliminary meeting it was formally resolved:

1. 'That in consequence of the above facts it does not appear incumbent on those who issued the circular and convened the meeting to proceed to Devonport.
2. That this meeting considered itself competent to establish the Association proposed in the circular.
3. That an Association be formed of the Medical Officers attached to Hospitals for the Insane whose objects shall be improvement in the management of such Institutions and the treatment of the Insane, and the acquirement of a more extensive and more correct knowledge of insanity.
4. That the Medical Gentlemen attached to Hospitals for the Insane be individually addressed and requested to join the Association.
5. That, by the members of this Association, the terms Lunatic and Lunatic Asylum be abandoned except for legal purposes and that the terms Insane person and Hospital for the Insane be substituted.
6. That to effect the great objects of this Association visits will be made annually to some of the Hospitals for the Insane in the United Kingdom, and that the order of rotation in which such visits shall be made be determined at the several meetings.
7. That the concurrence of the Governors of the several Hospitals to this arrangement be solicited by the respective Medical Officers.
8. That at its meetings the Association shall ascertain and record, as far as possible, the medical and moral treatment adopted in each hospital.
9. That to ensure a correct comparison of the results of treatment in each it is strongly recommended that uniform Registers be kept and that tabular statements upon a like uniform plan be circulated with the Annual Report of each Hospital, or where this be not practicable, that it be otherwise transmitted to the Association.
10. That at the meetings papers and essays be read; subjects of interest to the insane and to the Association be discussed, and information communicated and that a copy or minutes of these be preserved in the Journal of the Association.
11. That at the Annual Meetings the Senior Medical Officer of the Hospital visited be the Chairman.
12. That a Secretary be appointed to keep the Journals, papers etc. of the Association and to perform the usual duties of such office.
13. That the first annual meeting be held at Nottingham early in the month of September next of which due notice shall be given.

14. That Dr Hitch be requested to act as Secretary, pro temp.
15. That these Resolutions be printed, and a copy forwarded to every Medical Officer of the Hospitals for the Insane in Great Britain and as far as practicable to the Medical Officers of similar establishments on the Continent.'[2]

Thus the Association was born. Accounts of the initial annual meetings are now given in some detail to provide a picture of how the Association functioned in its earliest days.

Annual meetings

1841

The first annual meeting of the Association was held at the Nottingham Asylum on 4 November 1841. Eleven members were present plus three asylum governors who attended as visitors (it was resolved that the governors of institutions where the association was invited to hold its meetings should be invited to attend). It was also agreed that future members should be proposed by two existing members, the proposals should be sent to all members and a majority of two-thirds would be required for admission. The annual meeting would be held on the first Thursday in June of each year. The Association also decided that '[g]entlemen, whether medical or otherwise, who shall have distinguished themselves by their particular interest they have exhibited in the subject of insanity'[3] could be elected as honorary members. On this occasion, Mr Tuke of York, Mr Farr of London, Dr Bowden of Hanwell and Dr Ghislaine of Ghent were elected honorary members. Dr Shute was elected treasurer and with Dr Hitch, Dr Caselli and Mr Thurman formed a committee 'to consider the best form of Registers and tabular reports' as recommended at the Gloucester meeting.

It was decided that plans should be collected by and for the Association of all hospitals for the insane and that they should consist, as far as possible, of elevations, ground plans, sections, drains, etc. They should be accompanied by descriptions of the sites, soil, neighbourhood, etc. and reduced to a scale of 40 feet to an inch. They recorded that 'without pledging themselves to the opinion that mechanical restraint may not be found occasionally useful in the management of the Insane the members here present have the greatest satisfaction in recording their approbation of, and in proposing a vote of thanks to those gentlemen who are now engaged in endeavouring to abolish its use in all cases.' It was also requested of the chairman to express to the Secretary of State the opinion of the meeting that 'for the benefit of the insane poor' the word 'dangerous' should be omitted in the 45th Section of the Poor Law Amendment Act, when that measure shall be again introduced to the Honourable Members of the House of Commons.

---

2   Online archive 28. Association and College rules and charters.
3   Quotes, unless stated otherwise, are from minutes (handwritten), available from the College archives.

It was agreed that the annual subscription to the Association would be one guinea to be paid in advance of each annual meeting.

1842

The second meeting of the Association was held at the Lancaster County Asylum on 2 June 1842 when ten members and three visitors attended. The method of electing members was simplified to election by ballot at each annual meeting. Three acting members and two honorary members were elected. Plans for the Gloucester Asylum were received and Dr Crommelink of Bruges presented his Nouveau Manuel d'Anatomie Descriptive et Raisonnée. It was agreed to print his paper for distribution to members.

After that a letter describing the present diet in the Dundee Lunatic Asylum was considered – it was proposed to reduce the diet and the Association was asked for opinion. The meeting resolved,

'that as insanity is usually associated with a depressed state of the vital powers, and as experience has satisfactorily demonstrated the advantages which result from a liberal and increased diet in many of the larger institutions in the Kingdom for the insane, this Association conceives that any intention of reducing the supply of nutriments to the patients in the Dundee Asylum, whether in point of quantity or quality, would be extremely hazardous, inasmuch as the dietary at present in use, more especially as regards animal food, is already much below the standard in similar Institutions.'

Expressing their thanks to the visiting justices of the Lancaster Asylum, the members noted

'their great gratification at the improvements which are now in progress, but could not but lament that there is so small a quantity of land applicable to the employment and exercise of the patients – circumstances which experience proves to be so closely connected with the comfort and restoration of the Insane – more especially as the building is surrounded by a quantity of waste land admirably adapted for the purpose.'

They also agreed that the form for keeping registers of patients be adopted and the secretary be authorised to have it printed and a copy distributed to each member of the Association.

1843

The third meeting was held in London on 1 to 6 June 1843. It started at the British or Morley's Hotel (the Trafalgar Square) and the members were invited to visit four establishments (Hanwell, St Luke's and the Surrey and Kent asylums). The daily attendance varied between five, eight and twelve people. It was noted that the governor of Bethlem had refused admittance to the Association in the manner and for the objects described to them. Still, they 'entertained a hope that on some future occasion they may yet have the patronage of that celebrated establishment in addition to that of others in which their applications had been more favourably received.' Dr Pritchard was appointed auditor to the Association to report on its finances to a future meeting. A circular was to be sent to all members informing them that in future no annual subscription would be required from them and requesting an early payment of subscriptions now due for the past two years.

The secretary reported that 5000 copies of the register had been printed. He had also established a way of exchanging the reports and other documents of the hospitals for the insane in Great Britain for those in Europe and America. He had started a collection of British reports for the Association and hoped to have a full series by the next meeting. He also reported that in a correspondence between himself and Lord Shaftesbury on matters connected with the insane he had introduced the Association and offered its cooperation, which was accepted, and much useful information on the role of intemperance in producing insanity had been collected.

The secretary had – 'at the solicitation of several Medical Gentlemen connected with the Irish District Asylums' – addressed the government on the lack of a resident medical officer in establishments containing from one to 400 patients. The meeting approved of Dr Hitch's activities and recorded their opinion that 'nothing can be more detrimental to the comfort and welfare of the Insane than confiding the entire superintendence of Asylums to those who are not members of the Medical Profession.'

The secretary had had much correspondence on the amount of provision for the insane poor, and the impossibility of procuring this so long as the law for erecting lunatic asylums is 'permissible' and not 'peremptory'. The meeting concurred with observations in the letters concerning the importance of a more general and systematic provision for the insane poor and emphasised that attention should continue to be given to this subject with reference to probable legislative enactment. A plea for inserting a clause in any new Act of Parliament empowering the visitors of governors of county hospitals for the insane to grant retiring pensions to the officers was not supported by the Association. Two ordinary and fifteen honorary members were elected. Dr Oliver of Carlisle presented a paper, *Expediency of a General Method of Recording the Morbid Appearances met with in the Dead Bodies of the Insane*.

The meeting adjourned three times in the week to visit further institutions. The papers which the Association wished to print and distribute were read and further honorary members were elected including three clergymen, two of whom were chaplains. A letter was read which drew attention to the value of creosote in doses of three minims and upwards in cases of dementia where it seemed to have yielded good results. Another member wished to record the success of his use of opiates but omitted to state the circumstances and the quantities under which they were used. The meeting resolved itself into 'a conversazione on the respective experiences of the members in various forms of disease occasioning or accompanying Insanity.'

The meeting finally discussed the term 'matron' as the designation of the female head of hospitals for the insane. They noted that this was considered as highly objectionable in all cases, but more especially in those institutions where the patients were of different classes, and some of these of the higher class of society, from its associations with the female director of a workhouse. It was proposed to recommend a change in this but the meeting thought it prudent 'not to involve the Association by any expression of an opinion on the subject, but suggested that, in the cases where it appeared to operate most offensively, the Medical Officers should use their efforts to induce their respective committees to make the required alteration in the name.' This was the first meeting where the combination of the administrative matters, an attempt to collect statistical information, the delivery of medical papers and visits to local asylums had all occurred. With a less formal conversazione between members exchanging their experiences it was also the start of the social activities of the Association. This was to be the pattern of annual general meetings for the future.

1844

The fourth annual meeting was held at the Retreat, York, on 26 and 27 September 1844. One honorary member and three visitors were present. Dr Stewart of Belfast was appointed secretary pro tem because of the unavoidable absence of Dr Hitch whose report was read to the meeting.

A letter was received from Dr Julius from Berlin, drawing attention to the formation of a similar German association and stating that they would present a copy of the first number of their recently published journal. The German association also expressed the wish that both associations should publish a periodical devoted to the same subject and thus establish an exchange of publications. The medical superintendent of the Clonmel Hospital for the Insane (also known as the Clonmel Asylum) in Ireland sent his paper on the general management of the Irish district hospitals. It was recommended that this be brought to the attention of Lord Shaftesbury and the other Metropolitan Commissioners in Lunacy with an annexed statement as made to the Association by a member, of 'palpable imperfections in the existing management of the above Institutions and the utter want of any adequate provision for conducting the medical and moral treatment of their unhappy inmates, the medical officer charged with the same being a non-resident in all those establishments except one.' Further papers were read on homicidal mania and the use of opium and narcotics in acute mania. Hospital plans were also presented and Mr Tuke of the York Retreat discussed hospitals for the insane generally as buildings, 'making several valuable and practical observations connected with such Institutions particularly with reference to their Construction – Accommodation – Ventilation – means of Classification – proper number of patients sleeping together in the same room etc.', which were 'respectively heard with the greatest interest and attention'.

In its earliest formative years the Association depended on the energy of its first secretary who suggested rules, drafted plans, made proposals, organised the printing and circulation of papers, kept minutes and was responsible for all arrangements.

1847

The Association did not meet in 1845 or 1846 as they did not manage to find suitable venues and next met at the Warneford Asylum, Oxford, in June 1847. Nine members and two visitors attended and 11 new members were elected. The secretary had established an exchange of reports with American asylums and asked that the members should forward at least 40 copies of the reports of their respective asylums as soon after their publication as possible so that the exchange might prosper. He had received several plans of hospitals and the meeting resolved that a copy of each should be obtained and published by the Association and then circulated, in lithograph, among the members. Those members who had not submitted a plan would be urged to do so. They would also seek plans from the inspector of lunatic asylums in Ireland and would endeavour to obtain plans of the Clonmel Hospital for the Insane.

Mr Samuel Gaskell[4] read a paper on the construction of lunatic asylums in which he advocated a separation and detachment of the buildings instead of having one large and continuous structure. The meeting agreed with him and it was recommended that he should publish the paper in one of the medical periodicals and allow it also to be appended to the volume of plans proposed for publication by the Association. It was also recorded that the members were much impressed with the kindness and ability with which the Warneford Asylum was run and Dr Stewart of Belfast was asked to act as secretary to the Association for Ireland. Finally, it was resolved to periodically issue a volume of contributions relative to insanity and to psychology. The secretaries were authorised to communicate with members to ascertain how far they would contribute to such a publication.

There were no meetings in 1848, 1849 and 1850. One reason for the difficulty in holding yearly meetings was that railways were still in an early state of development and it was easier to attend a meeting in London than in an isolated provincial asylum. The first two meetings in London (1843 and 1851) were the only ones where over 20 members attended.

1851

The next meeting took place at the Freemason's Tavern, London, on 17–19 July 1851. By then the recorded membership had grown to 60. The 25

---

4 In February 1849 Mr Gaskell was appointed to the office of the Commissioner in Lunacy and in 1886 the Association approved the founding of a Prize Essay in his name (Online archive 36. Prizes and prize winners).

present, and a further 14 who were not there, were voted new members. Dr Stewart, secretary for Ireland, acted as secretary to the meeting. Dr Hitch resigned from this post, possibly because in five out of the ten years of the Association's existence it had not been possible to hold an annual general meeting, nor had there been much response to his circulars. He agreed to continue as treasurer. The secretary reported that he had endeavoured to carry out the directions of the previous meeting but regretted that they had accomplished little. They had received no additional hospital plans and their attempts to collect contributions for a published volume had failed entirely – no replies to the Association's resolution had been received.

After a discussion of current problems and difficulties caused by the Lunacy Acts (1828, 1845) it was resolved to form a committee to examine these Acts and to draw up a report, indicating ambiguities and defects, and suggesting alterations and amendments. The report would then be circulated among the members of the Association and presented to the Secretary of State and to the Commissioner in Lunacy. The committee, the first formal one to be set up by the Association, consisted of eight members, with Dr Forbes Winslow acting as secretary.

Dr Conolly, the chairman of the meeting, read an extract from a letter from Dr Williams of Gloucester recommending a petition to Parliament for the establishment of a Central Criminal Asylum and noting that such an asylum had been established in Ireland and was found to work admirably. Dr Conolly mentioned the 'unfavourable position in which criminals were now placed if the plea of insanity was admitted – their doom being actually worse than transportation and almost worse than death.' After further discussion of the arrangements in Ireland it was unanimously resolved that 'it is desirable that there should be a Central Asylum for Criminal Lunatics in England, distinct from any Asylum in which the insane, not criminal, are received. Dr Williams be requested to prepare a petition to this effect.' The government's decision that in future only qualified and experienced doctors should be appointed resident superintendents was welcomed. It was agreed that in future the Association would meet annually in London at the Freemason's Tavern on the second Saturday in July. Dr Aldwyn of Nottingham then exhibited and explained an improved lock-button for the purpose of securing the dress of the insane.

1852

In 1852 the Association met in Oxford and 15 members attended. Mr Ley proposed the establishment of a journal. Dr Bucknill addressed the meeting at considerable length on the issue and was supported by Dr Conolly. It was finally resolved to proceed with the journal and Dr Bucknill was appointed editor.

There was no meeting in 1853 but the first six issues of the *Asylum Journal* had been published, appearing at two-monthly intervals. After the first two years it was renamed the *Asylum Journal of Mental Science*, shortened to the *Journal of Mental Science* in 1858, a title it retained for the next 115 years.[5]

1854

Although it had been proposed that the Association should meet in 1853 in Manchester, the next meeting took place in London at the Freemason's Tavern on 22 June 1854; 13 members attended. Dr Hitch resigned as treasurer and Dr Ley was appointed in his place. Dr Kintman was appointed as auditor following the death of Dr Wintle, who appears to had been carrying out this function informally. It was agreed that future notice of meetings would be given in circulars addressed to each member as well as in the journal and that the meetings should be chaired by the president for the ensuing year. This arrangement continued for the next century. It was also agreed that a list of members would be published annually in the journal and that a committee should be appointed to revise the rules. This committee would consist of the president, treasurer, editor, auditor and secretary and it would have power to add to their number. There was a lengthy discussion on the rules and practices of the Association and many motions and amendments were passed.

Six members were also appointed to a committee to observe proceedings in Parliament likely to affect the interests of members and the institutions with which they were connected. There was considerable discussion on the desirability of obtaining a character reference from the resident medical officer of the relevant asylum before engaging any attendant or servant who had previous service. Individual patients were discussed, as were post-mortem findings in two cases. It was agreed to establish a branch office of the Association in Glasgow. Dr Bucknill reported on the progress of the journal. He had had numerous letters which indicated that it was highly appreciated and he had received many original papers from members. It had a significant effect in increasing membership numbers and broadening the Association's influence, but it was not, however, paying its way.

1855

The 1855 annual meeting took place on 19 July at the Freemason's Tavern, London, and 26 members were present. Dr Lockhart Robertson was appointed secretary and Mr Browne of Dumfries was appointed secretary for Scotland. Dr Stewart was reappointed secretary for Ireland. During the year 1854–1855 the Association had 121 ordinary members. The proposed rules of the Association, drawn up by the subcommittee were discussed and adopted.[6] Members were encouraged to publish their annual reports in a uniform medium-sized book. The subject of domestic treatment of the

---

5   Online archive 6. John Bucknill.
6   Online archive 28. Association and College rules and charters.

insane was discussed and it was recorded that 'this Association views with extreme regret the condition in which many insane persons, not paupers, are detained by their relatives in what is called domestic care and this Association believes that legislative enactment is absolutely requisite which will bring all insane persons under official inspection.'

The Association again passed a resolution recommending that establishments for the care and treatment of the insane should have only experienced members of the medical profession in charge. In recording this resolution, Dr Seaton said that the Association should take every opportunity to show the government and the public that lunacy is the result of disease. The opinion prevailing at that time that lunacy did not fall into the category of disease caused medical men to be regarded as mere keepers of madhouses. He hoped that the term would in future be expunged from the English language and that the medical men now engaged in psychological science would be looked upon as protecting the highest branch of the profession. This resolution had arisen following a bill before the late session of Parliament with reference to the District Lunatic Asylum in Ireland. Dr Stewart (the Irish secretary) pointed out that for the past 10 years only doctors had been appointed to the management of asylums in Ireland, but nevertheless, as the law stood, 'the Lord Lieutenant might appoint his valet or his butler to the office.'

The meetings were concluded with a dinner, a tradition that continues to the present day. An account of the 1856 dinner was given in the *Derby and Chesterfield Reporter.*[7] This feast was mirrored by the dinners given in later years, though at that time there were possibly more toasts and Victorian oratory than would be the case today.

Steady progress

By 1856 the Association had settled down to a period of gradual progress with new members elected at every annual meeting and a steady increase in their total number. This was helped by the development of the Journal, which carried full accounts of all meetings and activities. In 1858 over 50 members attended the annual meeting in Edinburgh. The title of the Journal was then changed to the *Journal of Mental Science* and 30 new members were elected. The Morningside Asylum was visited, and a grand ball was held there. Two hundred inmates took part in the festival, and 'danced with the most wonderful sane propriety, decorum and grace, reels and quadrilles, (polkas, waltzes and mazurkas being properly forbidden within the walls of the Asylum)'.[8]

---

7   The Dinner (1857) *JMS*, **3**, 15–18.
8   Annual Meeting (1858) *JMS*, **5**, 100–102; also see online archive 23. Asylum dance.

19

1861

The annual meeting was held in Dublin, with 21 members present. The Association had been steadily growing in its membership and that year it comprised 176 members (including officers) and 22 honorary members. Six members were elected to the Committee of Management in addition to the officers, and the finances were checked as satisfactory (see Chapter 8).

Dr John Conolly was not able to attend, but in his letter of apology he drew attention to the need to watch for any changes in the law that might make it more difficult for doctors to treat the mentally ill.

'For two or three years past, we have in this country been kept uneasy by successive menacings of legislative interference; the truth being that, regarded as physicians engaged in the treatment of mental disorders, we are already impeded and degraded by acts of parliament drawn up, for the most part, by lawyers, without respect to medical opinions or the feelings of mankind. I feel extremely anxious that medical men practising in insanity should steadily keep this in view, and diligently watch any legislative efforts that may be reviewed.'

The anomalous situation in Ireland was discussed in detail – the resident medical officers were not in charge of the asylums they worked in. A resolution was passed that the medical treatment of the patients in public asylums for the insane could only be efficiently carried out under the superintendence of the resident medical officer. After the meeting a deputation visited at Dublin Castle the new Chief Secretary Sir Robert Peel, to draw attention to the anomalous position of the alienist physician of the Irish district asylums. Sir Robert promised to give his immediate and best attention to the several important matters brought before him.

The following year, when the meeting was held in London, the Irish members were anxious to acknowledge the firmness and energy with which Sir Robert Peel had dealt with the question of the position of the resident physicians in Irish asylums. He had done this with strength and persistence in the face of considerable opposition on the part of the Privy Council in Ireland. The rules he promulgated were assimilated as far as possible to those of England.

Sir Robert Peel acknowledged the Association's thanks for his efforts:

'I am in the receipt of your letter of the 2nd, and am obliged to you for the opportunity you have afforded me of giving expression, in less formal terms than can be conveyed in a dry official acknowledgement, to my warm appreciation of the unanimous approval by the superintendents of asylums in this country of the rules recently promulgated by the Irish Government for the better management of the District Lunatic Asylums in Ireland'.[9]

9　　Letters on Irish District Asylums (1862) *JMS*, **8**, 355.

1862

In 1862 Dr Bucknill was appointed Chancery Visitor by the Lord Chancellor and resigned as editor of the journal. A special meeting was held in September 1862 to elect him an honorary member and to appoint his successor. Dr Lockhart Robertson was appointed editor and Dr Harrington Tuke was elected secretary in his place.

1863

That year there was a lengthy discussion about the Bethlem Hospital which led to the Association passing the following resolution:

'That the members of the Association have regarded with especial interest the question of the removal of Bethlehem Hospital to a site more adapted to the present state of psychological and sanitary science, and affording enlarged means of relief to the insane of the middle and educated classes in impoverished circumstances, and that they desire to express their concurrence in the representations already made to the governors of that important institution by the Commissioners in Lunacy'.[10]

The question of having a library was also addressed (discussed in more detail in Chapter 14).

1864

In 1864 the Association again discussed the problems arising from the judge's answer in the case of Daniel M'Naughton and the following motion was proposed by Dr Tuke:

'That so much of the legal test of the mental condition of an alleged criminal lunatic, which renders him a responsible agent because he knows the difference between right and wrong, is inconsistent with the fact well known to every member of this meeting, that the power of distinguishing between right and wrong exists frequently among those who are undoubtedly insane, and is often associated with dangerous and uncontrollable delusions.'

There was considerable discussion on this, as described more fully in online archives.[11]

The Association would hardly have remained in existence from 1841 to 1854 without the enthusiasm of its founder and first secretary, Samuel Hitch. In 1852 John Bucknill was appointed editor of the journal. In the next ten years the number of members trebled. From small beginnings, the Association had increased in stature and influence, thanks mainly to the enthusiasm and persistence of its founder and to the establishment and growth of the journal which brought it to the attention of a wider audience. In 1864 the name was changed to Medico-Psychological Association (MPA).

---

10   Notes, News and Correspondence (1863) *JMS*, **9**, 434.
11   Online archive 25b. Forensic psychiatry.

Further reading

Renvoise E. (1991) The Association of Medical Officers of Asylums and Hospitals for the Insane, the Medico-Psychological Association and their Presidents. In *150 Years of British Psychiatry* (eds. G. E. Berrios & H. Freeman), Vol. 1 (1841–1991), pp. 29–78. Gaskell.

Walk, A. & D. L. Walker (1961) Gloucester and the beginnings of the RMPA. *Journal of Mental Science*, **449**, 603–632.

Early minutes (handwritten) in College archives.

CHAPTER 3

The Medico–Psychological Association

The early years (1866–1900)

The change of name to the Medico–Psychological Association (MPA) in 1865 marked a move towards a more professional organisation, working both for its members and for better conditions for the mentally ill. The *Lancet* commented favourably that the new name expressed its essential scientific aspirations and called, among other things, for a uniform plan of recording asylum statistics to develop the as yet inadequate knowledge base and further the study of insanity.[1] The main issues during this period (1866–1900) divided broadly into two categories: the first covered internal and professional matters such as the purpose and venue of meetings, premises, the widening of the membership (whether or not to include women and the non-medically qualified) and the provision of pensions and other domestic matters; the second was concerned with the care and treatment of the mentally ill, as this was a period in which many further asylums were built and the number of inpatients greatly increased, many of them having chronic illnesses of a variety of kinds.

Internal and professional issues

The period began appropriately with the presentation of a bust of one of the pioneers of the specialty. During the 1866 meeting held in Edinburgh a letter was read from Baron Jaromir Mundy, a regimental surgeon and honorary member from Bohemia, who presented the MPA with a bust of Dr John Conolly, one of the advocates of non-restraint of which Mundy was an enthusiastic supporter. He wrote:

'The bust of Dr Conolly which I have sent to you is executed by one of the most renowned Roman sculptors – Cavaliere Benzoni. Be kind enough to present it to the Association as a humble gift of mine on this solemn occasion. I leave it to you and to my dear friend Dr Maudsley to move, where – with the agreement of the Association – this memorial shall be placed.'[2]

The most appropriate site for the sculpture was discussed at length and it was eventually decided to present it to the Royal College of Physicians. The president stated that 'in presenting this bust to the College of Physicians,

---

1   The Medico–Psychological Association (1865) *JMS*, **11**, 441–442.

2   Annual Meeting (1866) *JMS*, **12**, 416–417.

not as guardians, but as possessors, we are placing it appropriately in the hall of that College of which Dr Conolly was so distinguished a member'.[3] Dr Monro suggested that a copy of the bust should be made and retained for the Association, 'having the double satisfaction of presenting it to the College of Physicians, and thus having it placed in a position of great honour, and also of having a memorial of Dr Conolly amongst ourselves'.[4] (This idea was noted but it was not until 1988 that the present author, then president of the Royal College of Psychiatrists, arranged to have a copy made to be displayed in the College premises. In 1994 the two Colleges agreed to exchange the busts and the original now sits in the board room in Belgrave Square.)

Since its inception, the Association had normally held annual meetings, mainly in London. In some years, the meetings were not held at all, but this changed from 1854 onwards and the Association met every year. In 1868 it was agreed that, in addition to the annual general meetings, there should be quarterly meetings for the purpose of scientific discussion. The first such meeting was held in London later that year in the premises of the Medico-Chirurgical Society; 22 members and 6 visitors attended.[5] The president, Dr Sankey, gave a paper on the state of the small arteries and capillaries in mental disease and Dr Harrington Tuke, the secretary, spoke on the history and purpose of the Association. Discussion was lively and the meeting was deemed a success. Quarterly meetings now became a regular part of MPA activities, the first four being held in London. The first one held outside London took place in the Royal College of Physicians in Edinburgh in November 1869 with an attendance of around 20 from all over Scotland and the north of England. Subsequent quarterly meetings were generally held in London, Edinburgh and Glasgow but there was a meeting in Manchester in 1871 and a special meeting in Dublin in 1872.

The possibility of acquiring premises rather than using those of other organisations and hospitals for meetings had been under discussion for some years. In 1893 the idea came to fruition when the association obtained its own rooms at 11 Chandos Street in London, in the headquarters of the Medical Society of London, an arrangement that lasted for the next 80 years (see Chapter 15, Premises). The secretary reported on the terms agreed:

'Until the completion of the alterations about to be carried out on the ground floor of the Medical Society's premises, the association has the temporary use of one of the bookcases at the rental of one pound per annum and the use of the library for Council meetings at one guinea a meeting and the large meeting room for ordinary members at two guineas per afternoon. These terms include the right of using the Medical Society rooms as the official address of the Association as well as permitting the Hon. Secretary to make occasional use of the library for the purpose of conducting his official correspondence.'[6]

---

3   ibid., p. 419.
4   ibid.
5   First Quarterly Meeting (1868) *JMS*, **14**, 587–590.
6   Annual Meeting (1893) *JMS*, **39**, 598.

The balance sheet for the year 1897 reveals that the amount of rent paid for the premises that year was £102 and 7s.5d.[7]

Amalgamations

At the 1869 meeting in York a proposal was put forward that the Association might unite with the Medico-Chirurgical Society – the future Royal Society of Medicine – which was to have seven sections, one being Psychological Medicine.[8] A committee was set up to consider this and report whether the resultant changes in organisation would be desirable and whether there would also need to be adjustments to the running of the Journal. The committee presented their report to the 1870 meeting, though there was a procedural problem in having it considered since it had not been put formally on the agenda.[9] In supporting its discussion, one member said that if they stickled so much for matters of form they would expend a great deal of time unnecessarily and his good sense prevailed. Two members of the committee were in favour of amalgamation, the rest firmly against. After protracted discussion, a resolution was proposed in the following terms: 'It is almost unanimously agreed by the Committee that the amalgamation of this Association with any other Medical Society is undesirable.' An amendment reading 'that the amalgamation of the association with the Medico-Chirurgical Society is not desirable' was finally carried by 13 votes to 8.

Widening the membership

This matter had been raised at the 1865 meeting when it was suggested that it might be possible to admit non-medical members to the Association.[10] It was finally agreed that the Association will 'consist of Medical Officers of hospitals and asylums for the insane, public and private, and of all legally qualified medical practitioners.' Honorary membership, however, could still be granted to some individuals who were not medically qualified but prominent in the field. It seemed to go without saying at this stage that membership was a male preserve. The issue was raised again in 1871 in a consideration of proposed alterations to the rules, when the main question debated was whether to extend membership to include anyone interested in any way in psychological questions.[11] Henry Maudsley, as president, stated that if they were to admit members of that kind, they would be likely to get 'what I may call a very peculiar class of member ... persons who, to say the least, have peculiar views – Swedenborgians and spiritualists, and people of

7   Annual Meeting (1898) *JMS*, **44**, 877.
8   Annual Meeting (1869) *JMS*, **15**, 465–468.
9   Annual Meeting (1870) *JMS*, **16**, 448.
10   Annual Meeting (1865) *JMS*, **11**, 397–401.
11   Annual Meeting (1871) *JMS*, **17**, 445–446.

that class – some of whom have thought that they might enlighten us very much if they could come and read papers here.'[12] In the event, those present agreed an amendment that they should maintain their distinctive character by retaining the rule that any member of the medical profession with an interest in the study of insanity might be admitted. In one paragraph of the draft rules, the phrase 'every person' was used and the question was then raised as to whether this was intended to include women. The answer was a swift and predictable 'No' and the phrase was substituted with 'gentlemen'. (This caused problems in 1893 when the first woman doctor to become a member was proposed.) The issue of widening the membership was now firmly on the agenda. The matter came up again in 1872. It was noted at that meeting that there were already one or two members who were not in fact medically qualified – generally magistrates with an interest in lunacy – but it was decided to continue to restrict membership, with those existing exceptions, to medically qualified men.[13]

In 1879 the rules on membership were revised yet again. Honorary membership could be conferred on no more than three individuals a year. Candidates, who had to be proposed by three existing members, were to be drawn from among 'distinguished members of the medical profession, and others who are eminent in Psychology or in those branches of science that are connected with the study of insanity, or who have rendered signal service to the cause of humanity in relation to the treatment of the insane, or to the Association.'[14] Corresponding members were recruited from foreign physicians engaged in lunacy practice and residing abroad. They had to be proposed by four members and their number could not exceed 30 at any one time. The amended rules continued to ensure that women could not be admitted as they stated clearly that ordinary members should be 'legally qualified medical *men* [italics mine] interested in the treatment of insanity.' Candidates for admission had to be proposed by three existing members and secure three-quarters of the votes cast. It was to take further 13 years before membership was extended to include women, although by 1888 women doctors were sitting the examination for the Certificate in Psychological Medicine and appeared, without comment, on the lists of successful candidates.[15]

In 1893 Dr Conolly Norman of the Richmond Asylum, Dublin, put forward the name of his protégé Dr Eleonora Fleury. Dr Norman was an established member of the Association, was well regarded by his colleagues and became president in 1895 as well as editor of the Journal.[16] However, his proposal caused consternation in some quarters and there was a vigorous discussion. The president, Dr Lindsay of Derby County Asylum,

---

12   ibid.
13   Annual Meeting (1872) *JMS*, **18**, 455–469.
14   Annual Meeting (1879) *JMS*, **25**, 430–443.
15   Annual Meeting (1893) *JMS*, **39**, 599–601.
16   Online archive 10. Conolly Norman.

clearly supported the nomination, stating: 'I cannot see how in common fairness or on what valid ground legally qualified women can be excluded from membership if they wish to join the association on the same terms and subject to the same rules as men.'[17] Dr Norman pointed out that Dr Fleury was a paid official in a public lunatic asylum. Women were working in their profession and it was quite unrealistic to continue to deny them membership of the MPA. Dr Yellowlees of the Royal Asylum, Glasgow, agreed with him. The law had given women the right to practise medicine, the British Medical Association had admitted them and it would be 'unwise conservatism' to exclude them. It was too late for an amendment to change the rules in 1893 and this had to be formally proposed at the next general meeting. The amendment providing for the admission of women was finally passed by 23 votes to 7 and Dr Fleury was elected in 1894.[18] Contrary to the fears of some who had opposed the idea, she did not 'impose her presence' at any annual meeting. She was absent from the 1895 Irish Divisional Meeting when her paper *Agitated Melancholia in Women* was read by the president[19] and she remained a member until 1924. Without doubt, her election paved the way for other women, and by 1900, 14 women were or had been members, including Dr A. Boyle, who became the first woman president in 1939[20]. In general, by 1900 the number of members grew to over 600 from 198 in 1861.

Superannuation

The concerns expressed for many years with the problem of pensions are a good example of a profession looking after itself. In 1864, the Superannuation Committee had submitted a memorandum to the Commissioners in Lunacy, in which they stated that 'no settlement of the superannuation clause will be found satisfactory which does not – as throughout the military and civil services of the Crown – confer the retiring pension as a matter of right.'[21] The 23rd meeting (1868, London) saw a debate on this increasingly contentious issue.[22] The current arrangement was that a pension could be granted after 15 years of service and could be set at two-thirds of salary and allowances. The issue was that this was by no means universally applied and had now come under the administration of the Quarter Sessions rather than the Committee of Visitors for each asylum. The MPA was anxious that their members should receive a pension as a right and to a standard formula, and the president had brought to their attention the superannuation clause of the Lunacy Acts Amendment

17   Lindsay, J. M. (1893) Presidential Address. *JMS*, **39**, 480.
18   Annual Meeting (1894) *JMS*, **40**, 687–697.
19   Irish Divisional Meeting (1895) *JMS*, **41**, 547–555.
20   Online archive 10. Conolly Norman.
21   Memorandum on Retiring Allowances (1864) *JMS*, **9**, 610–612.
22   Annual Meeting (1868) *JMS*, **14**, 406–408.

Act 1862 on which he had written to the Commission in Lunacy. On 14 February 1868, the Commission replied:

'Adverting to possible legislation this Session on the subject of Asylum Superintendents' pensions, I am directed by the Commissioners to inform the Committee of the Medico–Psychological Association, that this Board feels that the opposition in Parliament to the claims set forth by the Association in their last published resolution on the subject would be quite insuperable. The Commissioners, desirous of supporting as far as possible the interests of the Superintendents, propose simply to seek an excision of the Statutory proviso which now renders confirmation by the Quarter Sessions necessary to any valid grant of superannuation. Should the Committee, after this communication, desire to press their views upon the Commissioners, it is requested so to do without delay. A meeting of the Board takes place on Monday next, at 12 o'clock, and would afford an opportunity of discussing the matter which may not again occur in time for legislation this Session.' [23]

The president, Dr Lockhart Robertson, reported that he and the honorary secretary had attended the Board at the time specified but that there seemed no hope in the short term of Parliament agreeing to the proposal of pensions as of right. The Commissioners, however, had invited the Association to send them a memorandum on the question to try to find an acceptable solution. The memo was duly composed and included examples of unequal and unjust operations of the existing superannuation arrangements in the county asylums, including the sad case of Dr Lawrence who retired in 1867 from the Cambridge asylum 'utterly broken in health' and was granted an allowance of only £50 a year for 12 years. Dr Lockhart Robertson asked the Commissioners to revert to the previous method of deciding superannuation, which was at the discretion of the Committee of Visitors rather than by the Quarter Sessions as had been decreed by the Lunatic Acts Amendment Act in 1862 and which was resulting in very arbitrary and varied decisions. The matter rumbled on without resolution but it was by no means forgotten. It was certainly on the agenda in the South-Western Division in 1898 when Dr Macdonald pointed out that, 18 months earlier, the asylum superintendents of England and Wales (with the exception of four London superintendents) had signed a petition in favour of compulsory pensions.[24] It was agreed to appoint a small committee to consider the details and formulate a scheme for the next meeting with a view to submitting this to Parliament.

This was one example of the MPA acting as a trade union for asylum medical officers. Those concerned were anxious that they should be treated in a fashion similar to those working for the government in the army or colonies of the British Empire. The pensions question was not in fact resolved satisfactorily until 1909 when the Asylum Officers' Superannuation Act became law, thanks in large part to the dogged persistence of the Association in keeping it constantly before the relevant Parliamentary committees.

---

23   ibid.
24   South-Western Division (1898) *JMS*, **44**, 633–638.

Care and treatment of the mentally ill

Before the 19th century the care of the mad was not always considered to be a medical issue. Mentally ill people were a family responsibility, with private madhouses for those who could afford them and prisons, workhouses or public madhouses such as Bethlem, in London, for those who could not. The treatment given amounted to little more than purging or blood-letting, with the violent patients put under restraint. This gradually changed with the work of Pinel in France and John Conolly in England, among others, who promoted the idea of non-restraint and the establishment of public asylums, built by voluntary subscription. The Retreat founded by the Quaker Tuke family introduced 'moral management' of the insane, modelled on the ideal of family life where patients and staff lived and worked together in a calm but controlled environment.

The most important figure for British psychiatry in the 19th century was the Seventh Earl of Shaftesbury. Although he was strenuously involved in a wide range of charitable activities, a major concern for the whole of his life was for the mentally ill. He subscribed to the belief that care, kindness, moral treatment and the abolition of restraint would lead to cure in early cases of insanity. He was an admirer of Pinel, Conolly and other pioneers of the non-restraint movement. He was averse to the involvement of the law and magistrates in decisions about treatment and detention. By the 1870s Shaftesbury was satisfied with the progress made in the treatment of lunacy. He remained insistent on early treatment and non-restraint. He noted an improvement of the standard of attendants, both male and female, in asylums and the fact that they were also better paid. In 1885 he resigned the chairmanship of the Commission of Lunacy for a time because of what he described was his repugnance to the introduction of magistrates into the process of placing a patient under care and treatment.[25,26]

Place of care

By the mid-19th century there was growing concern about the provision and appropriate place of care for the insane. In its comment on the appalling state of the care of the insane, the *Lancet* hoped that their condition in workhouses would receive urgent attention:

'Whether a few old and harmless imbecile patients may not properly be left in the workhouses is not a matter of very great moment; but that it is entirely unjustifiable to keep in the workhouse for one hour longer than is absolutely necessary an acute case of insanity, any one who knows what are the requirements of treatment in such cases, and what workhouses at present are, must feel most strongly. It will be remembered that our commissioners, in the course of their inspection of workhouses, discovered such things as a patient

25   Online archive 5. Shaftesbury.
26   Hodder, E. (1886) *The Life and Work of the Seventh Earl of Shaftesbury*. Gaskell & Co.

suffering from recent acute insanity, whose treatment consisted of the ordinary diet of the house; the plain meaning of which is, that just at the period when there is always the best hope, and often the only hope, or recovery through proper treatment, the unfortunate patient was, through official apathy or official neglect, left to degenerate into hopeless madness and to become a lasting burden upon society. It would be impossible to pass too severe a censure on so grave, cruel, and foolish an injustice.'[27]

Another issue at the time was what was called the 'cottage system of treatment of harmless lunatics and idiots', where patients in Scotland were farmed out to local households in return for payment. Many of the concerns about this expressed in 1868 were very similar to those raised more than one hundred years later about care in the community. It was pointed out that great anxiety was already felt in many of the districts of Scotland at the gradually increasing number of pauper lunatics, and there was reluctance on the part of the ratepayers towards increasing asylum accommodation. It was strongly urged by many authorities that the 'cottage system' of treatment for harmless lunatics and idiots provided adequately against any further expenditure in adding to the Royal and district asylums.

Dr J.B. Tuke, medical superintendent of the Fife and Kinross District Asylum, drew attention to the drawbacks of the cottage system, making a number of salient points.[28] First, the supervision of patients boarded out with guardians was totally inadequate. They should surely require more supervision than those in asylums with medical superintendents and other staff, not less as was the case at the time. Second, it was extremely difficult to select patients suitable for boarding out:

'The class which is said to be best suited for such treatment is congenital idiots or hopeless imbeciles. It is well known how very difficult it is to prevent this class of persons from degenerating and lapsing into the most degraded condition, even under very favourable circumstances: how much more likely is this to occur when the lunatic is committed to the care of a guardian who reaps an absolute benefit from a board ranging between 3s.6d. and 6s. a week?'[29]

Third, the capability of the guardians, most of whom undertook the task to supplement a low income, to care properly for their charges had to be questioned. It took months in an asylum to train attendants to an adequate standard – 'how, then, is it to be expected that the poor labourer or artisan can at once be fitted to undertake the office for which experience shows special training is absolutely necessary?'[30] Tuke pointed out that in every district of Scotland there was a district lunacy board. In most districts an asylum had been built to cope with the most urgent cases, but around 28% of patients were still boarded in private dwellings with inadequate supervision.

27   The Medico-Psychological Association (1865) *JMS*, **11**, 441–442.
28   Tuke, J.B. (1868) Gheel in the North. *JMS*, **14**, 431–432.
29   ibid.
30   ibid.

He suggested that district boards should be authorised to exercise care and supervision of all their pauper lunatics in both hospital and community.

Concern was expressed that it was difficult to admit all acute cases that required care because of the overcrowding of existing asylums. In 1870, Robert Boyd delivered his presidential address on the care and treatment of the insane poor.[31] He referred to the large numbers of pauper lunatics in workhouses and noted that, in some workhouses, separate wards were set aside specifically for insane paupers. In the discussion that followed, Dr Maudsley expressed the view that the insane poor would not be as well cared for in a workhouse as in a county asylum.[32] The alternatives for chronic cases seemed to him to be threefold: build further asylums, enlarge existing ones, or board out, as in the Scottish model. Dr Davey, on the other hand, maintained that county asylums were not the place to admit what he described as 'poor incurable idiotic imbeciles'. In his view asylums should be used for cases of insanity that could be cured. His experience of what would now be described as bed-blocking by incurable patients in two county asylums in Hertfordshire led him to suggest to the management committee of Colney Hatch that they should build an asylum that would accommodate between 250 and 300 of the 'recent and curable', pauper insane. His suggestion was not well received by the committee but he followed it up with several letters on the issue to the *Lancet*. The Commissioners in Lunacy subsequently recommended the provision of establishments between asylums and workhouses. This was not quite what Dr Davey had had in mind but a step in the right direction. Subsequent discussion at that meeting centred on the desirability of early treatment of the insane which offered the best promise of cures and the problem of containing the vast number of people with chronic and incurable illnesses. One contributor suggested an early experiment in community care, with one county selected to turn all its lunatics out of the asylum and observe the results. Finally, a vague proposal was put forward and agreed to, 'to facilitate the early admission of all acute cases of pauper insanity into county asylums, by providing for the proper care and treatment of chronic and harmless cases elsewhere'.[33]

During much of the 19th century concern was expressed about private madhouses and asylums. Much of this was driven by fear that a person might be detained improperly in such a place, to the final benefit of the proprietor. At the same time, if they could afford the fees, the families of people with serious mental symptoms preferred their relatives to be treated or confined in private rather than county asylums where there was more privacy, less stigma and overcrowding, and less likelihood of having to associate with uneducated violent patients from the lower social classes. As the MPA membership included doctors from both private and public institutions there was always some tension between the two groups, but they nevertheless

31   Boyd, R. (1870) The Care and Treatment of the Insane Poor. *JMS*, **16**, 315–320.
32   Annual Meeting (1870) *JMS*, **16**, 458.
33   ibid., p. 465.

continued to meet together. Proprietors of private asylums were generally better off financially than the others and there was an incessant movement from the public to the private domain. Samuel Hitch, John Conolly and Henry Maudsley were three of the best known practitioners to have worked in public asylums early in their careers and later in private practice. An example of this tension and hostility can be found in a paper given by Dr John Bucknill, a former Lord Chancellor's Visitor, who had at one time been medical superintendent of a county asylum. He wrote that it was the duty of the medical profession,

'both collectively and individually, to strive that the pitiable and helpless class of diseased persons from whom the profits of private lunatic asylums were derived should not suffer longer than could be helped under the disadvantage of a worn-out old law. Sequestered as such persons had been from the professional care of those for whom he spoke, they were still, as diseased persons, proper objects of interest and regard, and medical men owed it to themselves and their profession, to see that the law which governed their care and treatment should be conceived and executed in the spirit of benevolence, of a scientific knowledge of disease, and of the true relations which the ethics of the profession taught as being consistent with the dignity and welfare of both medical practitioner and patient.'[34]

Dr Bucknill's paper was given at a meeting of the Metropolitan Branch of the British Medical Association, held at Bethlem Hospital on 21 January 1879, and there was further considerable discussion the following year. This was described in an *Occasional Note of the Quarter*, probably written by Dr Hack Tuke:

'The paper and the debate were alike what might have been anticipated – the former, able; the latter, the reverse of dull. No one could feel surprised that some irritation should be felt and expressed at so vigorous an attack upon the principle involved in the keeping of Private Asylums. The rejoinder was natural, and was forcibly put by Dr Hayes Newington in reply – the temptation to do wrong exists, but why should Private Asylum proprietors be supposed to yield to temptation more than any one else? To prove that in a certain calling wrongdoing may bring gain, and that men may be found who will so enrich themselves, is only to state what is unfortunately too true of any circumstances in which temptation and human nature are factors. The counter reply no doubt is that those who would suffer on the supposition of wrong being done are persons who are unable to look after their own interests, and are weighted by a foregone conclusion that their statements are unreliable. The whole force and vitality of the feeling which has been for some time aroused against these institutions lies in this fact. The public seem more willing to be guided by the theoretical objection, than by the absence of proof of considerable abuses existing in their practical working. We are satisfied of two things – paradoxical as they may seem to be – namely, that the general feeling of the community is strongly opposed to private asylums, and that the preference is generally given to them by the same community when

---

34   Private Lunatic Asylums (1880) *JMS*, **26**, 135.

the question of placing a lunatic under care arises. This preference is mainly due to the idea of greater secrecy in regard to a disorder to which a stigma is still unfortunately too often attached. We agree with the conclusion of the Lunacy Commissioners that private asylums supply a want that the public asylums do not exactly meet. As it is the friends of the patient, and not the patient himself who is the second party to the agreement with the physician, we hold that Parliament has a right to step in, if for good reasons it sees fit to interfere. In fact it has already claimed and exercised the right to interfere.'[35]

In his presidential address fo 1879, Dr Lush, proprietor of Fisherton House, a private asylum, had unsurprisingly supported the private asylums:

'Admitting the excellent management of the public institutions, I hold that there are, and ever will be, many who object to the quasi-publicity involved in them, and who will prefer the comparative privacy of Licensed Houses for their friends. There is undoubtedly an active although fractional party desirous of upsetting the present Acts, and the most vulnerable point of attack is found in the supposed interest of private proprietors in the reception and detention of unsuitable cases: but the true interest of a proprietor is in the reputation of his House, and with the present supervision and checks, the admission of improper cases is well nigh impossible; that is, if the same care and attention are bestowed upon Public Asylums by the Commissioners in Lunacy as my own experience teaches me they devote to private institutions; and that the tendency of the present system is in the direction of too early discharges. It is notorious that many Doctors refuse to sign certificates in the clearest cases, from dread of responsibility, and of possible future annoyance; the Press seems eager to publish sensational accounts of supposed unjust detentions; while magistrates and judges, with one voice pit the so-called liberty of the subject against the danger to the common weal, to the detriment of the latter; and with another refuse to accept the plea of insanity in a large number of cases where prejudice or obtuseness alone can fail to detect it, and so inflict punishment upon irresponsible victims. Projects for boarding out paupers, and for the demolition of licensed houses are crudely put forward; and in the haste for cheap philanthropy, their authors set aside all considerations for the national weal.'[36]

In subsequent discussion Dr Monro of Brooke House in Clapton referred to Lord Shaftesbury's contrasting evidence to the Select Committees of 1859 and 1877:

'In 1859 there was hardly a word bad enough for him to use about private asylums, but when he gave evidence before the Select Committee in 1877, one of his last observations was that so high was his opinion of private asylums, that if it should please the Almighty to impose such an affliction upon him, he hoped he might be treated in a private asylum.'[37]

The lunacy acts of 1889–90 (the Lunatics Law Amendment Act 1889 and the Lunacy Law 1890) did not, in the event, abolish private asylums, but they

---

35   Occassional Notes of the Quarter (1880) *JMS*, **26**, 71.
36   Lush, J. A. (1879) Presidential Address. *JMS*, **25**, 311–313.
37   Annual Meetings (1879) *JMS*, **25**, 311.

laid down that no new licenses were to be granted and encouraged county councils to make provision for private patients in their asylums.

The criminally insane

The relationship between medico-mental science and the administration of justice was a long-term concern to the Association. The issue was raised publicly in 1843 when Daniel McNaughten, a Glaswegian woodturner, had shot and killed Edward Drummond, Private Secretary to Prime Minister Sir Robert Peel. McNaughten had believed that he was being persecuted by spies and had gone to the police and various public figures seeking help. His delusions gradually focused on the Tory Party and Peel as its leader. In his trial at the Old Bailey, a defence of insanity was put forward on the grounds that he had suffered from delusions for many years. He was found 'not guilty by reason of insanity' and was admitted to Bethlem hospital. The verdict caused public outrage and was debated urgently in the House of Lords, at whose request the judges drew up guidelines, known as the McNaughten Rules, for future cases: 'To establish a defence on the grounds of insanity, it must be clearly proved that, at the time of committing the act, the party accused was labouring under such a defect of reason, from disease of the mind, as not to know the nature and quality of the act he was doing, or, if he did know it, that he did not know what he was doing was wrong.' The Rules never became law but were nonetheless accepted by the courts, although they were strongly criticised by many as providing a concept of insanity that was too narrow.[38]

The issue of the insane in prison was also on the agenda. At the 1865 meeting Dr Mundy referred to the report of the Commissioners of Lunacy in Ireland who had recently drawn attention to the fact that 500 patients were still in prison; he called on the meeting to censure this practice in the strongest possible terms.[39] In 1873 the Association looked at the parallel problem that arose from criminal lunatics being sent to county asylums and noted that there were more of them in such asylums than in the criminal asylum at Broadmoor. A committee was set up (the Criminal Responsibility Committee) to monitor the situation.[40] Difficulties between the medical and legal professions have continued up to the present day.[41]

The education and training of doctors

There was little formal teaching of doctors in asylums or medical students in universities, although the Association continually pressed for this. A

---

38   Rollin, H. (1996) Forensic Psychiatry in England: a retrospective. In *150 Years of British Psychiatry*, Vol. 2 (*The Aftermath*) (eds H. Freeman & G. E. Berrios). Athlone Press.

39   Annual Meeting (1865) *JMS*, **11**, 413.

40   Annual Meeting (1873) *JMS*, **19**, 477–479.

41   Online archive 25*b*. Forensic psychiatry.

notable exception was in Leeds, where undergraduates could attend lectures and demonstrations by James Crichton-Browne (later knighted) at the West Riding Asylum, Wakefield. Wakefield, Leeds and York, sometimes referred to as 'the Wakefield triangle', were the centre of psychiatric research in the latter half of the 19th century.[42]

James Crichton-Browne, born in 1841, initiated a scientific approach to the brain and its diseases in his ten years as director of the West Riding Lunatic Asylum at Wakefield. He converted the Asylum to a better staffed hospital with more medical nursing and lay staff, all financed by local government. He enforced necropsies as a routine and started a laboratory for anatomy, neuropathology and histology. He conducted trials of virtually all neuroactive medicaments. He insisted on proper records and in 1871 began publishing annual medical reports. These ceased, however, in 1876 when Crichton-Browne became Lord Chancellor's Visitor in Lunacy. In the same year he co-founded and co-edited the journal *Brain*. He was president of the Association in 1878 and died at the age of 97 in 1938.

Welfare and training of asylum attendants

At the 1877 annual meeting Dr Clouston read a paper the *Question of Setting, Training, and Retaining the Services of Good Asylum Attendants*.[43] He stated that at the beginning of 1875 there were 72 000 insane persons registered and under control and there were 6000 paid officials to act as their attendants (a ratio of one attendant to 12 patients). He stressed the importance of training new attendants, providing a rising pay scale leading to an adequate pension, encouraging *esprit de corps* among attendants and making them proud of their profession. A committee of three was then established to consider the advisability of the formation of an association for registering attendants.

In 1892 it was suggested that the Association compile a handbook for nurses and attendants, as the existing one needed updating. A committee was appointed to revise and publish the handbook under the authority of the MPA. In 1894 the registrar reported on the examination for the Certificate of Proficiency in Nursing, which was proving popular. There had been 356 applicants, but two had withdrawn; the remaining 354 came from 29 different asylums and included one man from a private asylum. The number of certificates awarded was 281. Altogether 787 certificates had so far been issued and one attendant's name had been removed from the register for reasons unspecified.[44] The Association continued to be concerned about the welfare and prospects of all those who worked in asylums and their efforts were rewarded by the passing of the Servants of Lunatic Asylums Act in 1897, which dealt with staff pensions. There was also a dawning concern about the aftercare of patients discharged from asylums. In 1879,

---

42   Online archive 8. Sir James Crichton-Browne.
43   Clouston, J. S. (1877) *JMS*, **22**, 662–666.
44   Examination for the Certificate of Proficiency in Nursing (1894) *JMS*, **40**, 705–707.

for example, the Association for the After-Care of Poor Persons Discharged Recovered from Asylums for the Insane was established, principally to help rehabilitate female patients back into domestic and social life.

Patients' views

Sociologists have noted that most histories of mental illnesses and their treatments, when written by psychiatrists, tend to concentrate almost entirely on the views of doctors, while the views of patients are heard less frequently. The views of patients treated in the Morningside Asylum in the last quarter of the 19th century have been described lately by Dr Allan Beveridge.[45] He reviewed those patients' letters which had not been sent but had been retained in the asylum and appended to the patients' case notes. The superintendent of the asylum was seen in many guises: he could be a jailer, an autocrat, a petty tyrant, a wise philosopher, a kindly physician, a friend, an enemy, a confidant, a spy, a lover, a foreboding patriarch, a money-grubbing madhouse keeper, a Christian, a heathen, a respected member of his profession and a low dog. Many upper class private inmates professed to regard him as their social inferior, while the pauper patients were more deferential. A lot of patients had expressed shock and surprise when they found they had been admitted to an asylum. They found the asylum day stultifying with its predictable and unchanging timetable of early rising, eating, exercise and early bed. Further, the asylum rules were puzzling. There were many letters from patients to their relatives asking to be released. They were aware that the medical assistant's future could depend on the physician superintendent. Attendants might be regarded as merely keepers or prison guards; the most common complaint against them was that of using physical force. Many patients found the most disturbing feature was the other residents. Many believed they should never have been in the asylum at all as they were not insane and they frequently blamed their relatives for their detention. Dr Beveridge's review of letters written over three decades gives a telling and insightful analysis of how patients saw themselves, the institution and their personal predicament.[46]

Theories about mental illness

The masturbatory theory of insanity

A theory that masturbation led to mental illness prevailed for a surprisingly long time. Eighteenth-century physiology had taught that the vital fluid which was the flame of life dwelt in the semen, thus seminal loss consequent

---

45   Beveridge, A. (1998) Life in the Asylum: patients' Letters from Morningside, 1873–1908. *History of Psychiatry*, **9**, 431–469.

46   Online archive 20. Patients' views.

on compulsive masturbation was regarded as peculiarly depletive. A Swiss physician, Samuel Tissot, who believed that masturbation was very dangerous, had one of his books was translated into English as *Onanism or a Treatise upon the Disorders produced by Masturbation*. It became widely believed that this activity could be a precursor to insanity. Many alienists accepted this idea and endeavoured to prevent masturbation, sometimes in ways that seem appalling today.[47]

In his influential book *The Physiology and Pathology of Mind* (1867) Maudsley wrote that self-abuse:

'will produce an innervation of nervous element which, if the exhausting vice be continued, passes by a further declension into degeneration and actual destruction thereof. The habit of self abuse notably gives rise to a particular and disagreeable form of insanity characterised by intense self feeling and conceit, extreme perversion of feeling and corresponding derangement of thought in the earlier stages and later, by failure of intelligence, nocturnal hallucinations and suicidal or homicidal propensities.'[48]

At the 1876 annual meeting Dr Yellowlees described his method of treating masturbators, who were of all cases 'the most obnoxious':

'He had tried this mode in a dozen cases, and so far as it had gone he was very much satisfied with the results ... What he had done was to deal with the prepuce at the very root of the glans, to pierce it with an ordinary silver needle, the ends of which he tied together. He had the case of a lad who was so extremely addicted to masturbation that his mother begged him to do what he could to prevent it. He used the apparatus first in the case of this boy, with most excellent results. He had been masturbating night and day, and he was now so well that he was working as a carpenter ... The sensation amongst the patients themselves was extraordinary. He was struck with the conscience-stricken way in which they submitted to the operation upon their penises. He meant to try it upon a large scale, and go on wiring all masturbators. The moral effect of it in the house was excellent, and one man was seen weeping over his in anticipation of its disablement.'[49]

Dr Robertson responded,

'If anything can be suggested to prevent patients from practising this vile habit, which is the cause of insanity in many cases and aggravates the disease, it would be of very considerable importance. We know various things have been tried previously, such as blistering the penis, croton oil &c. but without effect: and various medicines are given with the view of moderating or repressing the desire. Dr Yellowlees' experience is short; but so far as it has gone it promises to be successful. We shall be interested to hear the result of these cases. Should they continue to prove beneficial in repressing this habit, I have no doubt we will all be glad to try it.'

47   Hare, E. H. (1962) Masturbatory insanity: the history of an idea. *JMS*, **108**, 1–25.
48   Maudsley, H. (1867) *The Physiology and Pathology of Mind*. p. 258. Macmillan.
49   Masturbation (1876) *JMS*, **22**, 336–337.

By 1895 Maudsley's views were modified, probably in response to the continental psychiatrists such as Kraepelin: 'Mental disorder due to self abuse is not always to be distinguished from simple adolescent insanity for the early symptoms of both are the same and are due to the processes of adolescence and not to the particular vice.'[50]

Treatments

It was thought that the early asylums would prove curative for the mentally ill and that failure to treat or cruel treatment in inauspicious surroundings would lead to deterioration to an untreatable chronic state. It was hoped that early transfer to a clean and safe environment with good food and attention would help nature to restore the disquieted mind to normality. Some of the public asylums followed the example of Tuke at the Retreat and tried to treat patients without recourse to restraint, but others felt that this was impossible to achieve.

During this period there were no specific drug treatments for any of the mental conditions seen. Examination of the presidential addresses reveals that by the 1870s, leaders of the asylum doctors remained sceptical of the efficacy of chemotherapy, such as it then was. In 1871, Maudsley, for example, expressed considerable caution: 'It seems to me that we are yet grievously in want of exact information with regard to the real value of sedatives in the treatment of insanity ... in all cases my aim is to dispense with sedatives as far as I can; and it often seems to me that the patient begins to improve when he begins to do without them and not in consequence of them.'[51] Many doctors stressed the importance of moral treatment in the management of the mentally ill, while the value of the newer drugs such as bromide was doubted. Also questioned was the effectiveness of other treatments such as electricity, the Turkish bath and the wet pack. There were some concerns about the side-effects of many drugs then in use. Diagnosis remained incomplete and unsatisfactory since there was little firm understanding of the causes and underlying pathology of the various illnesses. But this was beginning to change. The first 'drug' treatment introduced for which there was a rationale was the treatment of myxoedema with thyroid extract. In 1874 Sir William Withey Gull recognised and described the disease that then became known as Gull's disease. Myxoedema, arising from a shortage of the hormone thyroxine, caused physical changes – increase of weight, skin changes, frontal balding – and mental changes in the form of sluggishness, depression and other symptoms sometimes called 'myxoedematous madness'. One of the early methods of treatment was to fry sheep's thyroid glands and eat them with currant jelly or brandy. In the 1890s treatment with desiccated thyroid extract began and the first patient to be successfully treated in the UK was recorded in 1891.

---

50   Maudsley, H. (1895) *Pathology of Mind* (2nd edn), p. 399. Macmillan.
51   Maudsley, H. (1871) Insanity and its treatment. *JMS*, **17**, 330–334.

Intemperance or inebriety

From the 1870s, excessive and uncontrollable drinking was beginning to be recognised by some as an illness leading to addiction or dependence and there was increasing awareness that alcohol could cause long-term and short-term physical and mental changes. But there was also a strong feeling, illustrated by the temperance movement that this was wickedness rather than illness. Clouston, for instance, looked on 'inebriate asylums as an unfortunate attempt to coddle drunkenness and patch up a wide and fruitful social mischief'.[52] As there was a lack of unanimity within the MPA as to whether alcoholism should be considered as a moral vice or a medical condition, the Association did not put forward a public view on the issue.

Asylum statistics

In 1864, the Association had established a committee of three – Dr Lockhart Robertson, Dr John Thurnam and Dr Henry Maudsley – to compile a series of tables and a form of register as the basis of a uniform system of asylum statistics to be submitted to the Commissioners in Lunacy for their approval. The committee, reporting in 1865,[53] drew attention to the fact that this idea had been discussed 23 years earlier when a form of register had been adopted at the annual meeting in Lancaster in 1842. It had, however, been superseded by the registers of admissions, discharges and deaths which became required by law and their suggested register had never been generally used. They were in no doubt that the use of the register would provide much fuller and more useful statistics than those provided by the

---

Box 3.1 Tables for compiling asylum statistics

I   Number of admissions, re-admissions, discharges and deaths by gender, with average numbers of residents in the current year.
II The same information as in Table 1 (defined above), but for the entire period of the asylum's existence.
III History of the annual results of treatment since the asylum opened.
IV History of each year's admissions to show, for example, how many of those admitted in a given year have been discharged as cured, died or remained in care x years later. (Table adapted from the Somerset Asylum Reports. Useful in regard to the vexed question of the increase in insanity)
V   Causes of death. (Adapted from the reports of the Commissioners in Lunacy for Scotland)
VI Length of residence in the asylum of those discharged as recovered and those who have died during the year.

---

52   Clouston T. S. (1876) The relations of drink and insanity. *JMS*, **22**, 265–270.
53   Annual Meeting (1865) *JMS*, **11**, 402–408.

legal register but they were not prepared to recommend the printing of a revised second edition of the original register at considerable expense unless a sufficient number of members 'pledge themselves to its adoption and use.' The committee felt that asylum statistics could be divided into three categories – medical statistics, financial statistics and domestic statistics, and recommended that, for the moment, the Association should confine its attention to the first of these. Six tables were suggested, as summarised in Box 3.1.

The committee stated that the introduction of these few simple tables into all asylum annual reports would be very helpful in creating the main facts required for statistical comparison and would not be a difficult task. Their use would not preclude the collection of other data by the various medical superintendents who wished to record more, but would at least provide a uniform core of information. They recommended their adoption by all members and attached to their report forms for the six tables, the form of register accepted by the Association in 1842 and a copy of a paper by Dr Robertson on a uniform system of asylum statistics, which had been read at the annual meeting on 5 July 1860. While the report was 'unanimously adopted', like many of the other earlier recommendations made by the Association, only a limited number of asylums provided the suggested tables.

Further reading

Renvoize, E. (1991) The Association of Medical Officers and Hospitals for the Insane, the Medico-Psychological Association and their Presidents. In *150 Years of British Psychiatry* (eds. G. E. Berrios & H. Freeman), Vol.1 (1841–1991), pp. 29–78. Gaskell.

Turner, T. (1991) Not with Powder and Shot. The Public Profile of the Medico-Psychological Association 1851–1914. In *150 Years of British Psychiatry* (eds. G. E. Berrios & H. Freeman), Vol.1 (1841–1991), pp. 3–16. Gaskell.

CHAPTER 4

The Medico–Psychological Association

The later years (1901–1925)

The first quarter of the 20th century was a period of consolidation for the Association both centrally and in its committees and divisions. Membership grew slowly from 616 in 1901 to 673 twenty years later, largely because of the First World War. In 1909 the Asylum Officers' Superannuation Act was finally passed, the successful culmination of 60 years of effort to obtain adequate pensions for MPA members. The proposal to apply for a Royal Charter was taken forward and it was granted in 1926. There were the beginnings of specialisms following the opening of separate hospitals or colonies for the mentally subnormal, and discussions about eugenics were current. Malarial treatment for general paralysis of the insane (GPI) was introduced, the first successful treatment for a major mental illness. There was increasing use of educational and recreational forms of therapy as well as psychotherapy and psychoanalysis. The effectiveness of the asylum system for the care and containment of the mentally ill and the status of psychiatry itself were continuing to come under close scrutiny. The Maudsley Hospital was opened, which brought about a new era in the specialty in terms of research, treatment and education.

Committees

In May 1901, a special committee – the Rules Committee – was appointed to consider the reprinting of the rules, the addition of amendments that had already been made and the introduction of other amendments as deemed necessary. This committee reported to the 1902 meeting held in Liverpool, when it was decided that a new committee should reconsider the matter after referral to the divisions. A new constitution was approved in 1903 with a number of key features:

- appointment of a Nominations Committee
- audit of Association accounts by two members outside the Council
- registration and publication of attendances of officials for two years
- fixing the dates of all general and divisional meetings a year in advance
- devolution of more power and interest to the divisions.[1]

---

1   Annual Meeting (1903) *JMS*, **49**, 755–770.

Much of the Association's work was carried out in committee and reported back to council and the annual meetings. A number of committees became permanent or at least renewable, while others, set up for one specific purpose, were disbanded once they had made their report. Some of the MPA committees in the early 20th century were the Parliamentary Committee, the Rules Committee, the Statistical Committee, the Educational Committee, the Library Committee, and the Tuberculosis Committee.

The Parliamentary Committee at this time was largely concerned with the ongoing pensions question and with reform of the use of the Lunacy Act, especially to give more protection to 'medical men giving certificates'.[2]

The Educational Committee reported on the new Nursing Examination which was regarded as much more satisfactory than the old one, and on the Certificate in Psychological Medicine for Doctors in which interest was flagging and which was seldom taken. The Library Committee discussed whether reviewers for the *Journal of Mental Science* should be allowed to keep the books sent to them for review. Opinions on this were strongly divided and the matter was resolved, at least temporarily, by a decision to wait for the editors' report. The report of the Statistical Committee was submitted to the 1904 meeting. This was an important milestone in simplifying and improving the compilation of statistical information to make it useful and relevant with four groups of tables – admissions (separating first admissions and readmissions), discharges, deaths and the residue of long-stay patients – and a Medical as well as a Civil Register.[3] The Commissioners in Lunacy had given their provisional approval to the scheme.

Conditions of service

The career prospects for a junior or assistant medical officer in the public asylums were poor and their conditions of service were unsatisfactory. They were expected to live in the asylum and remain single – even if they had been allowed to marry, the stipend they received would hardly have allowed them to support a family. They could hope eventually to become a medical superintendent with a much increased salary, a house, marriage and the senior administrative post. However, this was far from a guaranteed progression. It is not surprising that for much of its life the Association was concerned about terms and conditions of service and enhancement of pension rights. Its efforts were finally rewarded in 1909 when the Asylum Officers Superannuation Act was passed. When it became law the following April, it made asylum employment more attractive, especially for married men with families. and retirement with a pension at the age of 55 was made possible.

---

2   Notes and News (1907) *JMS*, **53**, 845–846.

3   Adjourned (1904) Annual Meeting (1905) *JMS*, **51**, 799–856.

At a quarterly meeting dinner after the passing of the Act, speakers waxed eloquent about the success of their efforts and everyone involved was thanked effusively[4]. The president, Dr Bevan Lewis, summed up the occasion as 'one of the most auspicious in the history of the Association ... It was a considerable achievement, the culmination of years of careful planning and effective advocacy.' The bill had been introduced by Sir William Collins MP as a Private Members' Bill, 'notoriously difficult to pilot through both Houses of Parliament.' As such, its sponsors were forced to accept a large number of amendments in the House of Lords to prevent the Bill being wrecked by the government.

Subsequently, psychiatrists, who were classified as 'mental health doctors', were entitled after 20 years of service to count each year as two for pension purposes. This meant that after 30 years in the service, their pension entitlement was for 40 years. This anomaly survived the birth of the National Health Service (NHS) in 1948 and only ended in 1995 when pension rights were finally standardised across the whole of the NHS.

Apart from remuneration and pension concerns the Association was aware that for assistant and junior medical officers there were few opportunities for teaching and research, or for keeping up-to-date with medical practice, because of the lack of out-patient clinics and the isolation from general medical hospitals. In 1911 a committee was appointed to consider this and review the reforms necessary in the training and service of assistant medical officers. The committee presented an interim report to the annual meeting in 1913 which was adopted and submitted formally to the Association in 1914.

The problems identified in the report were divided into three groups:

1   Absence of proper provision for the early treatment of incipient and undeveloped cases of mental disorder.
2   Few facilities for the study and research in psychiatry.
3   The unsatisfactory position of assistant medical officers.

Proposed remedies included the provision of voluntary treatment with clinics in universities, medical schools and general hospitals, and facilities for postgraduate education with asylum medical officers allowed study leave. It was also recommended that it should be possible for assistant medical officers to marry by the provision of sufficient remuneration and housing.

It was resolved that copies of the Report should be sent to the Home Secretary, the President of the Local Government Board, the members of the Board of Control, the Chairmen and Clerks of Asylum Boards and Visiting Committees, and the corresponding officials in Scotland and Ireland, and other persons interested in the subject 'at the discretion of the President of the Association'.[5]

---

4   Commemorative Dinner (1910) *JMS*, **56**, 174–183.
5   Annual Meeting (1914) *JMS*, **60**, 644–694.

The failure of the asylums

In the years leading up to the First World War the Association was increasingly aware that the over-optimistic assumptions of the previous century were not leading to the cures that had been hoped for. Removing those who were mentally ill from gaols and workhouses appeared to have achieved no more than their separation from criminals and other destitute members of society whose poverty was due to causes other than mental illness or mental retardation. Removal to a more salubrious situation, generally out of town, where warmth, food, cleanliness and some simple occupations were available did not lead to recovery. There were virtually no treatments of any value apart from good nursing for concurrent physical illness and little was known of the causes of mental illnesses. The new asylums were huge – often housing more than 2000 patients – but were nonetheless overcrowded. Staff as well as patients were highly regulated as is well illustrated by the 1901 Tooting Bec Hospital bath rules (drawn up in 1901 and still on the walls in 1961) and the Regulations and Instruction Book of the City of Cardiff Mental Hospital 1919.[6]

Once the public asylum system had become established, however, society was able largely to ignore the problem of mental illness, while asylum doctors remained a relatively stigmatised group in the eyes of their medical colleagues and the public. Two incidents highlighted the problems and concerns of the asylum system at this time. The first concerned the suitability of the actual asylum buildings, the second the probity of the management.

The Colney Hatch fire

In 1903 there was a fire at Colney Hatch Lunatic Asylum in New Southgate in north London, a large hospital for the pauper insane. The fire started suddenly in the early morning at the bottom block of five temporary wards housing around 330 patients and 40 members of staff. The wards had been erected on timber frames and were lined with matchboarding. The flames spread quickly in high winds through this unsuitable material and despite heroic efforts by staff and fire fighters, 52 people died. In the subsequent inquiry, blame was laid on the London County Council, who insisted that increasing demands for beds had made it necessary to erect temporary buildings. It was also clear, however, that the Home Secretary and the Lunacy Commission knew that such buildings did not meet their strict standards of construction, but had not forbidden their construction. The tragedy led to a reappraisal of the design of asylums and made the use of temporary buildings, such as those at Colney Hatch, unacceptable.[7]

---

6   Online archive 24. Asylum rules.
7   The Colney Hatch fire (1903) *JMS*, **49**, 322–323.

The Horton Asylum scandal

In July 1904 four employees of the Horton Asylum were convicted of conspiring to steal groceries and other items from the hospital stores. One of the defendants, Charles Morant, a clerk, made a statement in which he claimed that the system of bookkeeping at the asylum was extremely faulty. It was usual to get rid of overstock and he had seen barrels of lime juice and vinegar and a ton of granulated sugar poured down the drain. In these circumstances, he had seen no harm in taking some items for himself. He also alleged that a number of asylum officials had received money from contractors for giving them the business. Counsel for the prosecution described his statement as 'absolute moonshine.' The jury found all the accused guilty of conspiracy but added that, in their opinion, the Horton Asylum had been badly mismanaged and that those responsible for its administration ought to be investigated. In passing sentence, the judge stated that the gross mismanagement of the asylum enabled him to take 'a lenient view of the conduct of the prisoners' and added that 'there was no proper control of supervision in the asylum'.[8] One of the problems undoubtedly lay in the method of management in London County Council asylums, which differed from that in county asylums, where the medical superintendent was fully in charge of all staff and had ultimate authority in the running of the establishment. In the city council institutions, medical superintendents had no such authority and could be undermined by other asylum officials.

Effective and ineffective treatment developments

Malarial treatment for General Paralysis of the Insane

General Paralysis of the Insane (GPI), a usually fatal condition frequently found in the asylums, had been considered to be possibly caused by syphilis, though the fact that the standard mercury-based remedies had little effect led to some doubts if this was correct. The theory was finally accepted when spirochaetes, the cause of other forms of syphilis, were found in brain tissue. Subsequently, more effective treatments of syphilis were discovered in this period: first salvarsan, an arsenate-based medication developed by Paul Ehrlich and more effective for the early stages, and Julius Wagner-Jauregg's malarial treatment which could arrest GPI. The latter treatment sounds curious but it was found that raising the body temperature could kill spirochaetes in the brain. In 1922, after the end of World War I, British doctors visited Wagner-Jauregg's clinic in Austria to study his methods. Centres for malarial treatment were established in Britain, the foremost being the Horton malaria laboratory in Epsom, which was set up in 1925.

---

8   The management of the London County Council asylums and the Horton Asylum scandal (1904) *JMS*, **50**, 751–756.

Ten thousand patients were treated with a 30–35% recovery rate, which was a considerable advance. With the advent of penicillin to treat syphilis the disease became a declining threat and malarial treatment for GPI stopped in the 1950s. The laboratory at Horton, however, continued to be used for the study of malaria until 1975.

The Weir Mitchell treatment

Jean-Martin Charcot in France and Silas Weir Mitchell in the USA were among the physicians who made a serious attempt to treat patients with minor functional disorders or psychoneuroses. These were people with no apparent anatomical or biochemical organ lesion but who had symptoms such as anxiety, hysteria and obsessions. Charcot recognised the mental origin of these illnesses, but his treatment with hypnosis and suggestion frequently accentuated rather than cured the symptoms. Weir Mitchell believed that such morbid states were physical in origin and treated them accordingly, even though no one organ of the body presented any sign of disease. He observed that the patients were often thin, liable to sudden increases in heart rate, pale and sometimes anaemic. His theory was that they were suffering from exhaustion of the nervous system of a kind comparable to a rundown battery. They were easily fatigued, they had no energy to send to their stomach and so could not digest their food; their heart rate had become 'irritable' for the same reason. The lack of nutrition, which resulted from the failure to digest their food, increased the exhaustion, and a vicious circle was set up. Mitchell's treatment consisted of confining patients rigidly to bed; they were fed a special diet to increase their body weight rapidly; they were massaged so as not to become flabby; and they were isolated from their friends and from their business to have complete mental rest. However, critics pointed out that the patients were overfed and gained too much weight; they also claimed that complete isolation was not a good idea, and that massage increased the patients' irritability. T. A. Ross, a physician with experience of psychoanalysis, tried treating patients with the strict Weir Mitchell plan and initially achieved a remarkable success. When he began, he was enthusiastic and had good results. As time passed and he learned of relapses in old patients his enthusiasm faded. He found that even his immediate results were less satisfactory and when they became very bad indeed he abandoned the treatment.[9]

The phenomenon of early cures in the history of a treatment, with later gradually diminishing results, is common to many kinds of therapy, and similar treatment approaches intended to improve the mind by building up bodily strength had been used at earlier periods with no more satisfactory results. For example, the patients of D. T. S. Clouston in the Morningside Hospital, Edinburgh, complained of boredom, overfeeding and weight

---

9   Ross, T.A. (1923) *The Common Neuroses*. Edward Arnold.

gain.[10] Many years later the modified insulin treatment was advocated by William Sargant and Eliot Slater, with similar initial enthusiasm and later disappointment with the results (and also with gains in weight), leading to its abandonment.

The focal sepsis theory of mental disease

The focal sepsis theory with its associated practices was an alarming episode in early 20th-century psychiatry. This started with the work of Dr Joseph Cotton in the USA. He believed that the cause of much mental illness was an underlying physical illness from unseen infections and advocated the use of dental clearances and sinus washing to remove alleged foci of infection as treatment for psychiatric disorders. He went on to extend the search for sepsis, later recommending partial colectomies for, among others, manic depressives. Cotton, who was made an honorary corresponding member of the MPA in 1924, had visited Rubery Hill Hospital where Dr T. Graves was medical superintendent. Dr Graves (president of the Association during World War Two) became an enthusiastic proponent of this theory and concentrated on removal of teeth and treatment of oropharyngeal sepsis. The theory and its associated practices fell rapidly from favour in the 1930s because of lack of effectiveness and the development of other physical treatments.

Psychological methods of treatment

After the First World War psychological methods of treatment became to be used more frequently. Large numbers of soldiers were treated for 'shell shock' (the diagnostic label given to the soldiers' psychoneurotic and sometimes psychotic symptoms) which had been brought on by their experiences in the trenches on the Western Front. Special units were set up – for example the Maghull military hospitals near Liverpool and Craiglockhart (Scotland). Here soldiers were successfully treated at early stages of their illnesses using simple psychological methods. Other therapeutic measures included provision of congenial quiet surroundings and protection from disturbances, such as noises and the sight of the wounded, which would have been likely to evoke painful emotions and vivid memories. Many shell-shocked patients were irritable and childishly peevish and needed to be treated with sympathetic firmness, tact and insight. Some physicians considered isolation an appropriate method of treatment as the boredom it caused could sometimes work favourably, but it was also necessary to prevent the patient from dwelling upon his subjective troubles by occupying his mind with other things. Other treatments included suggestion and hypnosis, which could relieve many of the acute symptoms in early cases.

---

10   Beveridge, A. (1998) Life in the asylum: patients' letters from Morningside, 1873–1908. *History of Psychiatry*, **9**, 431–469.

Many doctors treating shell shock were familiar with the writings of Pierre Janet and Sigmund Freud and accepted that unconscious factors might play a part in the production of mental disorder. If cases were not treated soon enough rationalisation and systematisation of the feelings (anxieties, doubts, bad dreams, fears, nightmares, depression) could develop and other symptoms the patient experienced could become more firmly established. Discreet sympathy and tact on the part of a doctor who was endeavouring to discover something more of a patient's past mental history could reassure them, while a short and simple explanation of some elementary facts of psychology was often sufficient to bring about a major change in a patient's condition. Mental, like bodily, disorders needed to be treated early, but the organisation of psychiatric services before the War had precluded this. It was also pointed out during that time that shell shock involved no new symptoms or disorders, as all had been seen before in civil life.

Informal treatment

In the years after the War it was possible to move slowly towards voluntary admissions to mental hospitals as had been recommended in the Association's 1911–1914 report. Henry Maudsley, by now seen as a 'grand old philosopher', having become wealthy through his writings and private practice, worked together with Dr F. W. Mott from Claybury Asylum, to plan a new type of hospital. Mott was clearly the main engineer of the project, but it was in accordance with Maudsley's own ideas for providing for acute treatment, education and research in an institution linked with a university, very much on German lines. Maudsley was prepared to offer £30 000 to the London County Council for this purpose. The hospital, eventually named after Maudsley, finally opened with its research arm the 'Institute of Psychiatry' after the First World War. It was sited in south London, opposite the newly built King's College Hospital and could admit 'informal patients'. In the following 50 years it became a centre for research and teaching and led to the development of a cadre of well-trained, thoughtful, though sometimes sceptical, psychiatrists.[11,12]

Beginnings of specialisms

The first 25 years of the 20th century saw the beginnings of the development of separate specialisms within psychiatry. Special hospitals and colonies for those deemed to be mentally subnormal had been developed for many years and there had also been special hospitals for the criminal insane. An interest in disorders of childhood and the treatment of inebriety (later seen as a form of drug dependence) appeared.

---

11   Online archive 11. Henry Maudsley.
12   Online archive 12. Frederick Mott.

After the War the treatment of shell shock was further developed, with a greater interest in psychological methods, in such units as the Tavistock Clinic which furthered the psychoanalysis of Sigmund Freud. Some of the ideas and methods used at that time can be found in the forms of psychotherapy used today, such as the cognitive behavioural approach.

Towards a Royal Charter

The 25 years covered in this chapter were dominated first by the threat of war and then by its reality. During the First World War it was agreed that all the existing honorary officers would remain in post for the war's duration. The annual meetings were short and dealt only with routine matters. The Journal received far fewer submissions, as witnessed by the reduced size of bound volumes for this period. In common with medical colleagues in other specialties, many medical officers working in asylums were required to enlist in the armed forces.

Psychiatrists working in the asylum system were aware that they could be seen as less important than physicians or surgeons and also that the MPA was less esteemed than the medical Royal Colleges. For this reason they wished to promote the MPA and believed that the Royal Charter (and the term 'royal' in MPA's title) would help achieve this. The idea of applying for a Royal Charter had first been raised in 1890 when Dr Hack Tuke proposed that it was desirable. Their request was refused, and as an alternative, having failed to receive Royal recognition, the Association was registered as an Incorporated Association under the Companies Act (1862–1893) on 30 July 1895. After the War, as the Association's activities returned to normal, it was decided to reapply for the Royal Charter. This was granted in 1926 and the MPA duly became the Royal Medico–Psychological Association (RMPA).[13]

Further reading

Arieti, S. (1974) *American Handbook of Psychiatry* (2nd edn), Vol.1, p. 37. Foundation of Psychiatry.

Henderson D. K. & Gillespie, R. D. A. (1927) *Textbook of Psychiatry*, pp. 312–314. Oxford University Press.

Sargent, W. & Slater, E. T .O. (1944) *An Introduction to Physical Methods of Treatment in Psychiatry*, pp.148–156. E & S Livingstone.

Turner, T. (1991) Not with powder and shot. The public profile of the Medico-Psychological Association 1851–1914. In *150 Years of British Psychiatry*, Vol.2 (1841–1991) (eds G. E. Berrios & H. Freeman), pp. 3–16. Gaskell.

---

13   Online archive 28. Association and College rules and charters.

CHAPTER 5

The Royal Medico–Psychological Association

1926–1967

In 1926 the MPA was granted a Royal Charter and from the 1940s there were hopes that it would proceed to become a medical Royal College. Over this period the number of members increased dramatically, from 847 in 1931 to almost 4000 by 1971. During this time rational treatment of mental illness developed with the introduction of some useful drugs for the major psychoses and for severe depressive illnesses. There were also advances in the psychotherapies and treatments began to be evaluated using randomised controlled trials. At the same time misplaced therapeutic optimism led to the introduction of other treatments (some useless, some harmful), which were later abandoned. Academic psychiatry was growing further at the Maudsley Hospital and the Institute of Psychiatry.

The Charter Meeting

In 1926 the Medico–Psychological Association was granted the Royal Charter of Incorporation and the privilege of using the prefix 'Royal' with its name. The College of Heralds then granted a coat of arms, with the medical caduceus, the serpents of Aesculapius and the butterflies of Psyche. The acquisition of these status symbols was celebrated by an enlarged annual meeting in Edinburgh – the Charter Meeting – organised by Dr J. R. Lord, medical superintendent of Horton Hospital, Epsom, who had taken over as president following the death of Sir Frederick Mott. Dr Lord, or Colonel Lord, as he liked to be known – having been officer in command when Horton had been a war hospital – was a colourful, flamboyant personality. He was the most active member of the RMPA at that time. Not only was he the editor of the *Journal of Mental Science*, but he also took a large share of the work of the general secretary and, during his presidency, chaired the Research Committee and numerous subcommittees, in all of whose projects he took a hand. His presidential address was so long that after two hours he had to stop his delivery, but arranged for it to be published as a special supplement to the Journal of 78 pages;[1] many bound copies were distributed.

There was no Programmes Committee at that time, nor did the RMPA have a paid secretary or an office of its own. All preparations for the

---

1   Lord, J. R. (1926) The clinical study of mental disorders. *JMS*, **72**, 452–453.

unprecedently extensive meeting were, therefore, carried out from Horton with minimal assistance from other hospitals. Speakers presented papers or opened discussions on the topics of the day – encephalitis lethargica and its mental sequelae, educational psychology, psychoanalysis, preventive psychiatry, forensic psychiatry, and the malarial treatment of GPI.[2]

Treatments of the time

Attempts to treat mental illness more rationally burgeoned during the life of the RMPA. Dr Lord had been much involved in introducing malarial treatment for syphilis to England by developing the Malaria Laboratory at Horton Hospital (called the Mott Clinic). While many of the treatments used during this period can be criticised with hindsight, there was at least an effort to do more than simply confine or restrain the mentally ill and those with mental subnormality.

Recreational and occupational therapy

After the First World War the best form of treatment of mental illness was believed to be – and to a large extent still is – the removal or mitigation of its causes. When this was not possible, readjustment therapies were used to make the best use of the patient's remaining abilities. The re-education of the mentally ill was thought to depend upon the replacement of bad, perverted, peculiar, slovenly and unsocial reactions by habits that were social and conventional. Work began to be seen as a source of diversion for a disturbed patient and occupational therapy proposed a range of activities that could be used. These included arts and crafts which could calm an anxious patient or revive the interest of the retarded depressive patient. Tasks that would give the brain-damaged patients some degree of satisfaction were provided for them. The first UK school of occupational therapy was founded in 1930 by Dr Elizabeth Casson, a psychiatrist, at Dorset House, Clifton. Industrial therapy aimed to provide a patient with a working day, a regular wage and the prospects of working outside hospital. It gave a sheltered working environment for chronically ill patients where they could learn, practise and gain confidence in new skills. In some hospitals light assembly work began to be done with local firms, and after the patients had proved themselves, they could go out to work. Rehabilitation of people with chronic schizophrenia was always a difficult task. They needed graded tasks, much encouragement, careful assessment and supervision. These types of activity, which were a continuation of the treatment popular in the previous century, were the typical background to new treatments being introduced in mental hospitals.

---

2   Walk, A. (1976) The Charter Meeting 1926. *British Journal of Psychiatrists (News and Notes)*, **122**, 5–10.

Insulin coma therapy for schizophrenia

Deep insulin coma therapy, introduced in the 1920s in Austria, was very widely used for 30 years and was seen as the best treatment for schizophrenia in the English-speaking world.[3] It was popularised by the Board of Control (the successors to the Lunacy Commission) in England and strongly advocated by most of the senior psychiatrists and writers of textbooks in the UK. The theory behind the introduction of this technique was that insulin antagonised the normal effects of the products of the adrenal system which were viewed as the physiological cause of the schizophrenic illness. The treatment required a special unit and ample staff. Patients were given increasing doses of insulin on a daily basis till they went into a hypoglycaemic coma. This was terminated by the administration of glucose via a nasal tube or intravenously. Patients required continuous nursing supervision for the rest of the day since they might have recurrences of hypoglycaemia. The treatment continued for several weeks until there was a satisfactory psychiatric response or they had had 50 to 60 comas. The morning treatment and afternoon activities filled several weeks with close interaction and care. This was a change from conventional regimes where staff had to try and engage with withdrawn or contrary individuals with whom they had difficulty in empathising. However, there was a mortality rate of about 1% with this treatment and patients tended to become obese.

The professional consensus that deep insulin cured schizophrenia was disrupted by a 1953 *Lancet* paper, *The Insulin Myth*. The author, Dr Harold Bourne, pointed out that 'In most mental hospitals patients are given, at a conservative estimate, 50–100 times as much medical and nursing care, measured by the clock as the general run of non-insulin treated patients' and therefore that there was 'no sound basis for the general opinion that insulin therapy counteracted the schizophrenic process.' In response, many leading psychiatrists promptly sent condemnatory criticisms to the *Lancet*. However, a careful, controlled, randomised study at the Maudsley and Cane Hill hospitals found no difference at six months between those who had 'deep insulin' and a control group who had been given sodium amytal with recovery aided by dexamphetamine.[4] As by this time the phenothiazines had been introduced, deep insulin coma therapy was rapidly abandoned. It appeared that the positive effects that had been achieved with it depended on the enthusiasm of all concerned and the active rehabilitation programmes that accompanied the treatment.

---

3   Jones, K. (2000) Insulin coma therapy in schizophrenia, *Journal of the Royal Society of Medicine*, **93**, 147–149.

4   Ackner, B., Harris, A. & Oldham, A. J. (1957) Insulin treatment of schizophrenia: a controlled study. *Lancet*, **269**, 607–611.

Electroconvulsive therapy

Another treatment introduced in the 1930s was electroconvulsive therapy (ECT). This was an empirical treatment used to treat a condition (depression) without any rational explanation of how it might work. It had been observed and noted that occasionally severe psychological or physical shocks might result in recovery from mental illness, and drastic attempts to treat mental disease included anaphylactic shocks using injections of metal salts, foreign proteins, infective material, or animal blood. Electroconvulsive therapy, especially when modified in administration with anaesthesia, was less upsetting for patients but still effective. However, ECT was overused and misused; many patients considered it was not only a frightening experience but one that could have a detrimental effect on their memory. There was a continuing controversy about this and some groups of patients thought it should be banned.

Recent controlled trials suggest that ECT shortens the duration of recovery in severe depressive illnesses, particularly the delusional variety, though some of the improvement may be a placebo effect or possibly the effect of anaesthesia. Induced seizures have a profound but short-lived effect on brain function (acute organic brain syndrome) that affects performance in the rating tests by which mental disease is quantified. There is no evidence that these functional and biochemical changes affect specifically and fundamentally the underlying psychopathology of psychoses. In general, however, ECT (modified) is a relatively safe procedure. It has not been shown to be superior to drugs, though it may act more rapidly, but the side-effects of drugs are not negligible and can be serious. When used properly, ETC still has a small but important role to play in psychiatric treatment.

Prefrontal leucotomy

For many years some psychiatrists believed that operations that interfered with the prefrontal brain lobes had little adverse effect and might at times improve, rather than reduce, a patient's capacity for adjustment. In the 1930s, Egas Moniz introduced prefrontal leucotomy on the hypothesis that in mental disorders certain synaptic paths were controlling the abnormal behaviour patterns. The operation was developed empirically first by injecting alcohol into the subcortical white matter of the prefrontal lobes. Later a steel leucotome was used and cores of white matter were separated in the prefrontal area but not removed. The main effect of leucotomy was believed to be a reduction in the emotional concomitants of abnormal experiences, and in short-circuiting the ruminations that tended to accompany them. Initially, it was used widely in all types of severe mental illness, but later it was restricted to the treatment of chronic severe obsessional disorder accompanied by persistent tension and misery. Prefrontal leucotomy is seldom performed now, as more effective treatments appeared, and because its dangers and ill effects have been more fully appreciated. Psychosurgery can still be valuable but only in carefully selected cases.

53

Drug treatments

The successful use of drugs to alleviate some of the symptoms of mental illness was a major development in later psychiatric treatment. Despite the advances in treatment, it is salutary to remember Voltaire's views of doctors as those who pour medicines, of which they know little, into patients of whom they know less, to treat conditions about which they know nothing at all. This was true of virtually the whole of medicine in his day and remains partly true today.

Many drugs were used in psychiatry for their sedative effects, and often overused also by the general population, particularly for insomnia. Between the two world wars bromides had been widely prescribed for all minor nervous complaints and various neuroses, until it was then found that they could accumulate in the body, leading to chronic bromide intoxications (bromism). With the development of simple methods of measuring levels of bromide in the blood there had been a rapid change to barbiturates, which were thought initially to be totally safe and non-addictive. Two factors led to the demise of barbiturate prescribing: the discovery of drug dependency with severe withdrawal symptoms and an epidemic of sometimes fatal overdosing (with suicidal or other intention) by large numbers of people. Benzodiazepines then superseded barbiturates. They were widely trumpeted as a marvellous and safe alternative as it was very difficult to take a fatal overdose. At the beginning, they too were believed to be totally free of any possibility of dependence but it was then found that dependency could occur when they were prescribed over time even in small therapeutic doses.

Other drugs came in to therapeutic use in the second half of the 20th century which finally ceased to be used. One was LSD (lysergic acid diethylamide), which had been given experimentally by some psychotherapists in the hope of uncovering buried treasure in the unconscious mind, but this ceased to be acceptable when the drug began to be widely used, or misused, for social, educational or pseudo-religious reasons, and its after-effects became evident.

The final group of drugs that were very widely prescribed for a time were the amphetamines. These were used initially to treat a wide range of conditions such as depression and minor neuroses, but similarly their widespread misuse for hedonistic social purposes, together with their psychosis-inducing properties and stricter criteria for evaluating drugs in randomised controlled trials, led to their eventual withdrawal except in certain clearly defined special cases such as attention-deficit hyperactivity disorder (ADHD).

Antipsychotics and antidepressants

The effects of chlorpromazine in cases of schizophrenia were first described in 1952. This was an empirical discovery based on a chance observation. Promethazine, an antihistamine drug, was noted to have sedative effects, and chlorpromazine, which is chemically related to promethazine (both are

54

phenothiazines), was synthesised in the hope of increasing this sedative action. It was discovered, however, that its range of activity was wider, and it was soon being prescribed for a variety of conditions, particularly schizophrenia and mania.

Another chance finding was that patients with tuberculosis being treated with the drug iproniazid became rather more euphoric than might have been expected. It was suggested that if iproniazid had a mood-elevating effect, it might be related to its ability to inhibit the enzyme monoamine oxidase and thereby affect brain amine concentrations and that such compounds might be of therapeutic benefit in cases of depression. A variety of monoamine oxidase inhibitors that were less toxic than iproniazid were then developed and used successfully. Imipramine was synthesised in the hope of producing an iminodibenzyl derivative related to chlorpromazine with an even stronger sedative action. On clinical trial, however, imipramine had little sedative activity but exhibited antidepressant activity, and from this the range of tricyclic antidepressants was developed.

Lithium

Lithium carbonate was introduced following the confirmation of an earlier report that the element lithium was effective in improving the symptoms of mania. It later appeared to have a true prophylactic activity in preventing recurrences of both the manic and depressive episodes which occur in patients predisposed to manic depressive psychosis. Although lithium salts had been used in the 19th century for the treatment of gout and other disorders, they fell into disuse because of their toxicity. They were reintroduced for the treatment of psychiatric conditions in the 1950s following the experimental observation that lithium carbonate produced a short period of lethargy and unresponsiveness to stimuli in guinea pigs who, however, remained fully conscious. Lithium was considered to be of benefit in treating manic conditions, initially. It is now used in the prophylaxis and treatment of mania and the prophylaxis of bipolar disorder (manic–depressive disorder) and in the prophylaxis of recurrent depression (unipolar illness or unipolar depression). Lithium salts have a narrow therapeutic/toxic ratio and are not prescribed unless facilities for monitoring blood–lithium concentrations are available. Because of their toxicity the decision on the use of prophylactic lithium has to be based on careful consideration of the likelihood of recurrence in an individual patient and the benefit has to be weighed against the risks, with regular monitoring of thyroid function. The need for continued therapy has to be assessed regularly and patients should be maintained on lithium after three to five years only if benefit persists.

Two useless, now abandoned treatments

There was a remarkable surge of therapeutic optimism immediately after the Second World War. Treatments were developed with little or no rationale, flourished for a time and were then abandoned.

One unsuccessful treatment for psychoneurosis was the inhalation of carbon dioxide. The patient inhaled a mixture of 30% carbon dioxide and 70% oxygen. At the first treatment 20 to 25 respirations were given. After 8 to 16 respirations the patient usually lost consciousness and psychomotor excitement of various forms might be seen. Later, the lower extremities were slightly flexed and the hands showed carpal spasms (similar to the tetanic signs in hyperventilation). The pupils might become fixed, and a decerebrate rigidity-like state could develop. The number of treatments varied from 20 to 150. The theory behind the treatment was that psychoneurosis was caused by an abnormally low threshold of stimulation with respect to normal stimuli. The treatment was intended to raise the threshold of stimulation to the normal level of resistance to noxious stimuli from within or from without. Earlier reports suggested good outcomes but a subsequent controlled clinical trial concluded that the treatment had no specific therapeutic effect.[5]

Intravenous acetyl choline was introduced as a less drastic method of applying 'shock therapy'. Its most striking effect was apparent cardiac arrest for 30–50 seconds. The patient turned extremely pale after the injection and became unconscious. There occurred twitchings of the face and extremities and usually an extensive spasm. The use of acetyl choline never became widespread and later controlled trials showed no significant difference between those receiving acetyl choline and those on calcium glucamate (which produced sensations similar to those produced by acetyl choline).[6]

Fortunately, at the time as these new treatments were applied there was a significant progress in the methodology of clinical controlled trials, supported by advances in academic psychiatry developed at the Maudsley Hospital under the leadership of Edward Mapother and Aubrey Lewis.[7] Nowadays further research into drugs endeavours to find out which part of the drug molecule produces desirable or undesirable effects with a view to modifying and producing better and more effective drugs with less undesirable side-effects. Furthermore, processes occurring in the brain can be directly studied, for example using magnetic resonance imaging, which was impossible in the days when the Association was founded. Slow but genuine progress is being made.

Towards the Royal College

Following the Second World War and the founding of the National Health Service (NHS) in 1946 there were many changes in medicine. The introduction of more effective medication and other welfare reform led to a decline in the number of psychiatric beds needed. This led to Enoch

---

5   Hawkings, J. R. & Tibbetts, R. W. (1956) Carbon dioxide inhalation therapy in neurosis. *JMS*, **102**, 60–66.

6   Hawkings, J. R. & Tibbetts. R. W. (1956) Intravenous acetylcholine therapy in neurosis. *JMS*, **102**, 43–51.

7   Online archives 13. Edward Mapother & 14. Aubrey Lewis.

Powell's Hospital Plan in 1962, which envisaged closure of the large and by now decaying asylums, to be replaced by psychiatric units in general hospitals and community care.[8] However, revenues saved and capital from land sales were not necessarily directed towards the care of the mentally ill, nor were general hospitals or the community particularly welcoming. In parallel the function of the RMPA began to change and the role of physician superintendents to be questioned, along with that of asylums. The consultant grade developed, and the new consultants considered themselves to be equal to rather than responsible to the medical superintendents, rather to the chagrin of some of the latter.[9]

The idea of forming a Royal College of Psychiatrists first appeared in the minutes of the RMPA Council meeting held on 6 July 1948.[10] Dr A. Shepherd had written to propose that the Council examine the possibility of the formation of a college of psychiatry with authority to issue diplomas, memberships and fellowships. It was agreed that the officers of the Association should make preliminary investigations into this matter. It is not clear whether any action was taken at this stage but the issue appears again two years later in the Council minutes for the meeting on 11 July 1950 under the heading Proposed College of Psychiatry. On this occasion a resolution had been received from the Northern and Midland Division with regard to the establishment of a College of Psychiatry and the Council appointed a committee to investigate the advisability of this. The members of the committee were Dr K. K. Drury (president), Dr T. Tennent (treasurer), Dr R. W. Armstrong (general secretary), Dr H. V. Dicks, Professor D. R. MacCalman, Dr P. K. McCowan, Dr T. P. Rees and Dr W. Rees-Thomas. In November 1950 they recommended that the proposal for a medical Royal College should form the subject for discussion at the quarterly meeting of the Council in February 1951 and it was agreed that the afternoon session on 15 February would be devoted to this, with both those in favour and opponents to the idea invited to take part.

About 40 members attended the discussion, out of an approximate membership of 1250 – a poor representation. Professor MacCalman presented a strong set of arguments in favour of a medical Royal College and was supported by Dr Rees; Dr E. B. Strauss spoke against the proposal. The consensus was that no action should be taken at that time but that the proposal should be kept in mind and should be brought forward to the Council again in November 1952 and reviewed annually thereafter. The next time the matter came up was on 10 September 1952, when it was noted that there was no change in the position. At this meeting, however, it was first suggested that the Education Committee should be asked to consider the possibility of the RMPA, which was already an examining body, establishing

---

8   Tooth, G. C. & Brook, E. M. (1961) Trends in the mental hospital population and their effect on future planning. *Lancet*, **277**, 710–713.

9   Online archive 22. The penultimate medical superintendent.

10   Minutes, RMPA Council Meeting, 6 July 1948, College archives.

a higher qualification – a Fellowship – in psychiatry. Both matters were kept under review throughout the 1950s and towards the end of that decade there were informal discussions within the Royal College of Physicians of London about the possibility of creating a Faculty of Psychiatrists within that College.

In 1960 the RMPA Council discussed the matter once again and from this date on the issue remained more prominently on the agenda. A special committee set up in November that year to look at developments in psychiatry considered three possibilities:

- formation of a Faculty of Psychiatrists within the Royal College of Physicians
- retention of the RMPA with the creation of a higher qualification
- establishment of a Royal College of Psychiatrists.

The faculty idea foundered when it became clear that the physicians were unwilling to alter the regulations for membership to allow an examination run jointly by physicians and psychiatrists rather than just the former. The Royal College of Physicians of Edinburgh had already offered this concession to psychiatrists in Scotland but the London College was not prepared to be so accommodating and much psychiatric opinion in England then became set on achieving a separate Royal College of Psychiatrists. The attitude of the Royal College of Physicians was understandable. Historically they regarded themselves as covering medicine as a whole and were not keen to see this position fragmented. But as medical knowledge progressed, other specialties, such as pathology and psychiatry, could see their interests diverging and began to resent the domination of the physicians. The second possibility – retention of the RMPA with a higher qualification – was seen by many as a defeatist compromise and at this stage everything appeared to point towards the formation of a Royal College of Psychiatrists. There was not, however, sufficient support within the Council.

Further pressure to move towards founding a medical Royal College came from Dr John Howells and the Society for Clinical Psychiatrists (the former Group for the Representation of Clinical Psychiatrists).[11,12] It had been formed to press for equality between all consultant psychiatrists and medical superintendents wishing to remove the latter pre-NHS category. Dr Howells campaigned vigorously within the Association for a change to college status but was in a minority with the officers and Council against him. He, therefore, took his campaign to the membership starting a correspondence in the *Lancet* and the *British Medical Journal*. It continued from September 1963 to May 1964. Of the 67 letters printed, 49 were favourable to the idea of a medical Royal College and 18 against. In the meantime, the annual

---

11   Howells, J. G. (1973) The Society of Clinical Psychiatrists. *Bulletin of the Royal College of Psychiatrists*, 6–7.

12   Howells, J. G. (1991) The establishment of the Royal College of Psychiatrists. In *150 Years of British Psychiatry*, Vol. 2 (1841–1991) (eds. G. E. Berrios & H. Freeman), pp. 117–134. Gaskell.

meeting of the RMPA voted 85 to 26 in favour of a college, having previously voted by 70 to 64 in favour of holding a postal ballot of the membership. The Psychological Medicine Committee of the Royal College of Physicians (consultant psychiatrists who had also passed the Membership of the Royal College of Physicians examination, MRCP) voted 44 against and 5 in favour of a college. They also voted 23 in favour of a faculty of psychiatry but 21 were against. It had been suggested that the RMPA should take up premises within the new building of the Royal College of Physicians of London, but this would have increased their annual rent from £700 to £5000.

The Society for Clinical Psychiatrists circulated a questionnaire to their members and found that 74% favoured a college. They then sent the questionnaire to 1000 psychiatrists in Britain and found that 80% supported the idea. Dr Howells, having read the RMPA bye-laws, realised that after due notice he could raise any issue at an annual general meeting so he submitted a resolution to be raised at the meeting in 1963, advocating a petition for a Royal College of Psychiatrists. This was dealt with at the adjourned meeting and a postal vote was held in May 1964. The Society for Clinical Psychiatrists had circulated a leaflet encouraging all psychiatrists to vote; 68% did so and of these three quarters were in favour. Only 6% supported the suggestion of a faculty within the Royal College of Physicians. Although the postal ballot had shown a majority of members embracing the idea of establishing their own Royal College, it was still necessary to have the agreement of the general meeting before a petition for a supplemental charter could be drafted. Dr Howells sent a resolution to RMPA members advocating a College and preparing the ground for the annual general meeting in 1964. The Society for Clinical Psychiatrists sent a circular to members pointing out the importance of attending and the vote in favour of petitioning for a College was carried overwhelmingly by 150 to 9. Until this meeting, the officers and the majority of Council opposed the idea of a college, yet that changed. Dr William Sargant, the registrar, changed his views and became a supporter of the cause. On the other hand, Dr Alex Walk, the librarian who had done much historical research into the Association and had held most posts within it, remained of the opinion that the RMPA should not be changed at all.[13]

After the postal vote and the outcome of the meeting the Council set up a Petition Committee, which included Dr Howells and Dr Hutchinson from the Society of Clinical Psychiatrists, to start informal negotiations with the Privy Council on the form the petition should take. The negotiations took considerably longer than was originally expected as the Council decided to revise the bye-laws at the same time. Although theoretically it would have been possible to do no more than apply to have only the name changed to the Royal College of Psychiatry, this would in practice have meant no changes in the way the organisation functioned (as had previously happened in 1926).

13   Online archive 15. Alexander Walk.

Some members of the Petition Committee supported the suggestion that a Faculty be created and thought that the college should be modelled on the older medical colleges, particularly the Royal College of Physicians of London. The changes in the bye-laws were intended to enable this. However, there were two major problems to be faced. In the past, psychiatrists had been able to join the Association without taking an examination and other doctors could also join. The other medical colleges restricted their membership to those of the medical profession who had passed their entry examination. There was much discussion on restricting membership and introducing an examination. It was finally agreed to proceed in this manner and thus for the future membership would not be allowed to anyone who had not passed the new College's entrance examination. This meant that the ensuing negotiations lasted from 1964 to 1971 when the Supplemental Charter was finally granted.

CHAPTER 6

The Royal Medico–Psychological Association

1968–1972

During the final three years of informal negotiations with the Privy Council there was a growing concern among the RMPA membership about the form the college might take. Junior psychiatrists were particularly worried by the proposed examination and feared that the college would have little role in education and postgraduate training; they also expressed considerable anxiety about its future functions. In short, junior psychiatrists virtually revolted. The eventual remit of the college was significantly altered before the Charter was granted in 1971. The Council would initially have preferred the RMPA to become a faculty of the Royal College of Physicians, but Dr John Howells and the Society for Clinical Psychiatrists pressed for a College. The RMPA members gave their support and thus forced the Council to act. There were problems in transforming the Association which was open to all psychiatrists into a medical Royal College with strict entry criteria. The interest aroused, and the changes brought about, proved wholly beneficial in the long run, but at the time there was sufficient confusion and ill temper to make it an unpleasant period for most of those concerned.

Psychiatrists in training (and those who had passed one of the Diplomas in Psychological Medicine (DPM) examinations but had not yet obtained a consultant post) were concerned about the new college's membership criteria and an examination which all would have to pass to become its member, whether or not they were already a member of the RMPA. Such an entry examination was already in place for the other medical Royal Colleges (Physicians, Surgeons, Obstetricians and General Practitioners). The RMPA differed considerably from these Colleges in that it was an association which anyone could join, though full membership was restricted to psychiatrists. This meant that most non-consultant psychiatrists were members who received the Journal and could attend, and vote at, all meetings including the annual and quarterly meetings. Until draft proposals were circulated, they had not realised they would not automatically be full members of the college. There had been a steady increase in the number of members of the RMPA after the decision to become a College had been taken and it now was feared that one of the effects of the proposed examination might be that many psychiatrists would be kept out. (In the late 1960s at one point the probability of passing the physicians' membership examination on the first attempt was only 6%.) The general practitioners also had a limited membership since less than half the general practitioners in the country were members of their College and most saw the British Medical Association with its journal, divisions and meetings as their spiritual home. The second concern that began to be discussed was the lack of any adequate psychiatric training across most of the country. This led to a further suggestion that the proposed new college should be given the remit and the responsibility to ensure adequate teaching and training. It was this latter proposal that led the college to differ markedly, not only from the RMPA, but also from the older medical colleges. Inspection, vetting and control of postgraduate training were eventually included in the charter and the draft bye-laws of the proposed new college.

These developments came to a head in 1968 when doctors in training at the Maudsley Hospital raised their concerns, following much debate in the junior common room. Some supported the establishment of a faculty for psychiatrists within the Royal College of Physicians, others – the metamorphosis of the RMPA into a Royal College. These views changed over time when it appeared the London College of Physicians wished to restrict entry to the proposed faculty to those who had passed the membership of the Royal College of Physicians examination, albeit possibly with a part in psychiatry. Eventually, the physicians withdrew their objections to a psychiatric college. The discussions at the Maudsley then ceased to be about the pros and cons of a faculty or a college and became focused on the nature of the latter.

Trainees were worried that the proposals appeared to concentrate mainly on an examination, with little attention to teaching and training. Those at the Maudsley were aware that they were fortunate in their postgraduate education and that there were few centres which provided what they themselves were receiving. They drafted a letter emphasising that greater attention would need to be given to education and training schemes to ensure that junior psychiatrists were given an adequate grounding in the subject before they sat an examination. Many junior posts were isolated and most psychiatric units and mental hospitals had totally inadequate libraries. Most psychiatrists in training had no experience at all of child psychiatry, forensic psychiatry, subnormality or psychotherapy. Many juniors could spend several years doing the same work in an isolated hospital with no postgraduate teaching facilities. The letter was sent to the *British Journal of Psychiatry* and was initially accepted by the editor, Dr Eliot Slater, who later returned it saying that the RMPA Council did not think it should be published. The signatories then decided to send it to either the *Lancet* or the *British Medical Journal*, possibly stating that it had been turned down by the *British Journal of Psychiatry*. The two main points made in the letter suggested that senior trainees who had passed a Diploma in Psychological Medicine (DPM) examination should be exempted from sitting the entry examination and that proper education and training, rather than examination, should be emphasised as a criterion for membership.

A special Council meeting

This draft letter caused immense alarm within the Council. They appear to have taken the view that the Privy Council might now refuse to support the transition altogether, despite the previously universal agreement among psychiatrists themselves that this should be done. In an apparent moment of panic they decided to summon the signatories to persuade them to withdraw what they considered a damaging criticism. A special meeting of Council was convened on 8 June 1968. The president (Professor H. V. Dicks, a psychoanalyst) was abroad at the time and in his absence Professor Ferguson Rodger chaired the meeting as the most recent past president available. The letter was discussed and their Privy Council Agent voiced his belief that the publication of such a letter might postpone the possibility of the RMPA becoming a College. The Council took the view that there was no need to redraft their proposals as all the concerns could be dealt with in changes to the bye-laws after they had received the necessary new charter. They thought that a new College would not be acceptable to the Privy Council unless it was similar to the other medical Royal Colleges which had no entry except by examination. They thought the signatories of the letter lacked trust in the Council and its drafting and negotiating committee, and had to be a self-interested group who only wished to be exempted from the proposed new examination. The acting chairman supported this view, adding that the signatories must have been thinking at an unskilled-trade-unionist level, while using the as yet unaccepted arguments of the Todd report (on postgraduate medical education) to bolster their arguments.

The Council then invited representatives of the signatories to the meeting, which became unpleasant. They were hectored and treated discourteously and one member of the Council suggested that they could be expelled from the RMPA for their behaviour. A full account of this meeting is available in the council minutes.[1] This was not the reception the signatories had expected or deserved. It became known that the junior doctors felt they had been threatened by the Council. Some senior psychiatrists then joined them as their supporters. A so-called unofficial 'petition group' was formed to put forward a formal motion at the next general RMPA meeting. The most active members of this group were Dr Garry Low-Beer, Dr Angela Rouncefield and Dr Jim Birley (the Maudsley consultant), all of whom called for further action. There was also an open meeting at the Maudsley Hospital, when a correspondent from *The Guardian* was present, and so the problem became public and was widely commented on in the daily as well as the medical press. The petition group then circulated a letter among the RMPA members, giving their views and suggesting a draft petition which could incorporate training in the remit of the proposed new college. Their petition stated that 'in the assessment of general professional training there

---

1   *Special Meeting of Council*, 8 June 1968, College archives.

was no place for a single major "pass or fail" examination', which should be replaced by assessment 'on a progressive basis … Examinations should be seen as only one, and not necessarily the most important element in the assessment process.' Also, 'that over the period of its first five years the Royal College will take action to establish standards of training, and to promote regional training programmes of a quality such that, upon completion of their training, a high proportion of candidates would normally be expected to prove satisfactory.' And finally that 'the bye-laws be amended to allow that, for five years from the date of its inception, individual membership be granted to all candidates possessing a DPM, or equivalent qualification, and having undergone training satisfactory to the Royal College'.[2] It was unlikely that the Privy Council would agree to this since the entry to all the other medical colleges was by an examination.

The annual general meeting 1968

In order to ensure support for the motion a bus was chartered to take supporters of the petition group to Plymouth, where the annual meeting was being held. The president, Professor Dicks, chaired the meeting.[3] He had not been present at the special meeting of the Council and when the issue of expulsion threats was raised he initially endeavoured to deny that anyone had been threatened. There was then a lengthy discussion about this and the part of the Council minutes dealing with the encounter with the trainees was read out. Dr Noble (one of the signatories of the letter) then presented his impressions of that meeting. There were questions and a discussion between those present, as some of them felt they had been threatened with expulsion from the RMPA. There were also questions about the position of those who had signed the letter in relation to their membership in the RMPA, so the president asked Dr Skottowe to elucidate. Dr Skottowe reported: 'I asked, "Do you really mean that by sending a letter such as you propose you will be serving the best interests of the Association and if not would not the honourable course be to withdraw from the Association?" I never mentioned the word "expulsion."' The question of whether or not the word 'expulsion' had been used during the special Council meeting was further discussed, and a statement was made from the platform that it was believed that it had. The members were then assured that the use of the word was not intended to imply any threat to any member.

The general secretary then read the report of the Special (Petition) Committee which had met six times during the previous year. RMPA representatives and their agent had talked with the Privy Council Secretariat and they understood that any request that might be made for an interim

---

2   Papers relating to the work of the Petition Committee 1968–9, College foundation archive.

3   Annual Meeting (1968) *JMS*, **114** (suppl. Oct), 13–17.

period for admission of Foundation Members would not be granted; and that any suggestion to alter the standard for admission to Foundation Membership to less than consultant status in the health service, or its equivalent, would not be acceptable. The probable (indeed almost certain) effect of petitioning for any of these provisions would be the rejection of the petition, which could not then be presented again for five years at least.

This information made it clear that only three courses of action were possible:

- to accept what the Privy Council would require
- to petition for an interim period and lower standard of admission to Foundation Membership, or of examination, and have the Petition rejected
- to delay submission of a petition until the situation regarding the Royal Commission's Report (on medical education) and the Green Paper had been clarified.

In the light of this, the RMPA Special (Petition) Committee had recommended acceptance of those requirements that, after enquiry, they had reason to believe would be insisted on by the Privy Council. This report was received with applause.

There was a further lengthy discussion which led to the meeting being adjourned on a more conciliatory note. It was informally agreed that the junior doctors group (the informal petition group not to be confused with the Council's Special (Petition) Committee) might discuss with the RMPA legal advisor what might, or might not, be acceptable to the Privy Council, taking account of the concerns raised. A ballot was then taken on the original motion proposed at the meeting despite the junior doctors wishing to withdraw it. It was not surprising that there were 45 abstentions with 8 against the motion and 5 for it; this meant that all agreed to accept what the Privy Council would require. The meeting was then adjourned to allow time for the junior doctors' group to discuss how best to do this with the Council's legal advisors.

The reconvened general meeting[4]

This annual meeting in Plymouth (1969) was the critical moment leading to the major changes that came about. The outcome was that the College became a totally different organisation from the RMPA. Dr Pilkington proved to be a helpful and conciliatory president and it was following this meeting that there was a change of heart in the Council and the views expressed about training were taken on board and became part of the thinking of the RMPA. Some of the members of the petition group met Sam Silkin, acting as counsel for the RMPA, and found that the feared problems did

4 Adjourned Annual Meeting (1969) *JMS*, **115** (suppl. May), 1.

not exist and that there was no reason why the Court of Electors could not be given the authority to approve training programmes. The meeting was reconvened and met in London on 6 February that year. Two amendments to the proposed bye-laws were proposed by the petition group and were carried unanimously:

Membership is a mark of professional standing awarded only after a period of training and after examination, except for those medical practitioners who have attained an advanced level of professional experience and responsibility. Membership is a higher qualification which the possessor is entitled to use in self-description in a manner prescribed by Council so long as in doing so he does not imply that he is a Member of any other organisation. There shall be a Court of Electors charged with the duty of approving training programmes, carrying out the examination for admission to Membership, and electing to the Fellowship those qualified by bye-law 11; the Court shall be empowered to make the necessary regulations, subject to the overall control of Council. The Court may appoint subcommittees to carry out such parts of the above functions as it may direct.[5]

The president reported that he had had a fruitful meeting with representatives of the unofficial petition group, as a result of which the above bye-laws had been drafted. Dr Low-Beer, on behalf of the petition group, said how gratified the group were at the satisfactory conclusion to the discussions, and paid tribute to Dr Pilkington's handling of the meeting. It was the phrase 'the duty of approving training programmes' that made an immense difference to the way the new college would carry out its responsibilities when it came into being.

Although the question of oversight of training had been dealt with in the adjourned general meeting, the discussions about the future college had reached the press. On 1 September 1968, between the two RMPA meetings, for example, *The Economist* published an article entitled *Psychiatry – Who Wants to be Royal?* The author pointed out that although a previous ballot of the members of the RMPA showed a clear majority in favour of the transition to a college, a new radical group based mainly in the Maudsley Hospital and calling itself the petition group strongly denounced the examination proposals. They considered that a pass or fail examination ran quite counter to the recommendations of the recent Royal Commission on Medical Education. In place of such an examination the Commission had proposed a period of organised training and subsequent assessment and that membership and later fellowships of the college should be granted after this training. There were many similar articles in both the medical and general press with headlines such as 'Negotiational Threats'. For the next two years a bitter and rancorous debate continued with the arguments well and truly in the public domain. It did not cease even after the College formally came into being in June 1971.

---

5   ibid.

Association of Psychiatrists in Training (APIT)

On 22 August 1971 a group of psychiatric registrars and senior registrars from Birmingham, Edinburgh, Glasgow, London, Manchester and Sheffield met in Birmingham to discuss ways in which psychiatrists in training, as well as their seniors, could coordinate their efforts to express their needs effectively to the Royal College and to promote improvements in training throughout the country. At this preliminary meeting it was decided to canvass urgently, seeking nationwide support for the setting up of an Association of Psychiatrists in Training. A letter to the *Lancet* on 11 September that year (signed by 300 trainees) raised their questions about the new examination. Their letter ended:

'We wish to make it plain that we are not opposed to the concept of the Royal College nor to the idea of assessment including examination. We feel, however, that we must protest at this time about the form of this examination and we ask all junior psychiatrists to consider or reconsider their position about entering for the membership examination, particularly the first Part 1 in November, 1971, until the above questions have been answered. Because of a general feeling of unhappiness regarding the role of junior psychiatrists in the Royal College, an Association of Psychiatrists in Training is being formed.'[6]

Signed A. Clare and 300 other trainees

The *Lancet* commented on this in an editorial entitled 'College Capers':

'The Royal College of Psychiatrists came into being in June by transmogrification from the erstwhile Royal Medico-Psychological Association. So far the College has no president and no council; but it has circulated two documents setting out the provisional bylaws and the regulations governing its membership examination. It is the second of these that has prompted over three hundred trainee psychiatrists to sign the letter which appears this week. Our correspondents' concern is understandable. Nowadays most medical educators, even in the United Kingdom, concede that formal examinations as steps towards specialist appointments are on their way out, and that, pending their extinction, they should function as portals of entry to training rather than as passports to consultant status.

The Royal Commission on Medical Education – whose report every college should steel itself to exhume for occasional inspection – hoped that the early postgraduate phase would cease to be dominated by preparation for formal examinations, and insisted categorically that "in the assessment of general professional training there is no place for a single major 'pass or fail' examination."[7]

The College accepted this and started to inspect all trainees and training posts. In 1969 the RMPA itself jointly sponsored a conference in which the panel on assessment named as the first requirement of proposed

6   Correspondence (1971) *Lancet*, **298**, 598–599.
7   College Capers (1971) *Lancet*, **298**, 587–588.

examinations for psychiatrists' continuous assessment. An assessment on a standard form was to be made of each student's performance at the end of every 6-month period during their training. At that meeting Professor Martin Roth had said:

'We have a choice between the elimination at set intervals of a large and predetermined proportion of each cohort of students, which is unacceptable, and the admission, by a reliable criterion, of candidates who thereafter became the responsibility of the school. The teachers should then be expected to look after these men and in most cases guide them through their training to the end. Failure should be exceptional. I think it is very important that, once selection has occurred, the man should be almost certain of qualifying at the end.'[8]

The *Lancet* commented:

'Yet the College has decided on a two-part examination of which part I cannot be sat until at least three years after the start of training in psychiatry. If this examination were to be easy, it would be pointless. But it will not be easy, if only because the world must be shown that psychiatry has arrived as science – that the Smiths of Queen Anne Street are no whit inferior to the Joneses of Regent's Park. British doctors are resigned to the waywardness of the older colleges; but the Physicians at least have the grace to impose their membership examination at the start of training, where its harm is circumscribed, and not (as the Psychiatrists propose) near the end where it is calculated to prove the greatest nuisance, the greatest menace, and the greatest impediment to original work. The would-be psychiatrist will have to wait at least five years after graduating before he learns whether he is judged fit, by examination, to engage in his chosen specialty; and by then he will have given nearly four years' service in this specialty – years that for him will possibly turn out to have been fruitless, and will certainly have been warped by the prospect of the double hurdle that he must clear at the age of 30 or so. It may be questioned whether psychiatry lends itself to formal examinations at the beginning, middle, or end of training; and with any luck in a decade all membership and fellowship examinations will have been swept away by specialist board certification. Meanwhile the oncoming generation must face the facts of today; and one fact is that, barring some last minute intervention, the first primary examination for membership of the Psychiatrists' College is to be held in November.'[9]

This was an important event because membership was to be (in the words of the College's Journal) 'a qualification related to competence to practise at the level of consultant in the National Health Service.'[10]And apparently it would be the only such qualification if the College had its way. The *Lancet* pointed out that many senior psychiatrists who were members of the RMPA already examined for other bodies offering a psychiatric qualification such as the Diploma in Psychological Medicine (DPM):

---

8   ibid.
9   ibid.
10   ibid.

'Their services will now be available to the College, which cannot, of course, say what other examining authorities should do. Quite so. But how is the implied vision of the membership as the sole recognised qualification to be realised? An RMPA report on psychiatric education, issued less than three years before, described how a questionnaire had led to the conclusion that 'there is a substantial number of hospitals, recognised as providing experience for the [Diploma in Psychological Medicine] which are not meeting the most modest demands made by the Conjoint Board for this recognition, which allowed candidates from these posts to sit the Conjoint Board DPM. How, then, in this under-manned specialty, are enough training places to be found for the tougher membership examination? Perhaps the College hopes to force the more ill-equipped hospitals (which might otherwise find themselves short of staff) to raise their standards by installing a library, employing a psychologist, developing a programme in clinical psychiatry, and so on. But this will take time: in the interim how are the demands of the NHS for consultant psychiatrists to be met?[11]

Later that year the *Lancet* had a short leading article entitled 'A Speechless College':

'On September 11 1971 the *Lancet* published a letter, with over three hundred signatories, seeking information about the examination for membership of the new Royal College of Psychiatrists. The following week the College's interim president[12] said that there was an answer or a reason for each point raised in the letter and in an accompanying editorial; but that "This can come later." Since then a month has passed during which the College's Court of Electors has met, but as this issue went to press the College had vouchsafed no full response. It should delay no longer. The Association of Psychiatrists in Training, which owes its origin to uneasiness over the College's bearing towards junior colleagues, is to meet in Manchester on October 31. Before then the College should answer publicly the questions publicly raised in the letter. Failure to do so can only strengthen glum suspicions – that the answers are not quite so easy as the interim president suggested, or that the College is relying on time quenching the flame of incipient revolt, or that the College's acting officers are so deeply divided that they cannot agree on a common statement, or that they have taken a vow of silence until the College's first annual general meeting (in November 1971) has been allowed to pass in decorous outward accord. None of these possible reasons is at all creditable; and all become increasingly less credible with each passing day of silence. The College is not a club which potential psychiatrists can join or ignore at their pleasure: it is setting itself up to provide a qualification of competence to practise consultant psychiatry. In doing so, it has accepted an inescapable responsibility to explain fully the terms of the examination and to show convincingly that training resources match the requirements of this examination. So far the College has dismally failed to recognise, or at least to act on, this responsibility; and seemingly it still proposes to hold its first part-I examination in November. Any observer might be forgiven

---

11   ibid.
12   Martin Cuthbert, the last president of the RMPA, acted as interim president until the election of Martin Roth and his formal inauguration.

for concluding that behind the acquisition of the College's Royal Charter lies a right royal muddle.'[13]

At its meeting in Manchester on 31 October 1971, The Association of Psychiatrists in Training (APIT) backed a call for the temporary suspension of the membership examination to allow for consultation between all interested parties. They were considering boycotting the new examination and the College. In seeking such a suspension, the APIT claimed it was acting not with caution and that it was the Association that sought to prevent the College from prematurely committing itself to a course that could only be detrimental to the future of psychiatry. While the junior psychiatrists had made considerable progress in getting the new College to undertake responsibility for promoting training and had accepted the Privy Council's requirements on the criteria for Foundation Membership, much anxiety remained about the nature and timing of the qualifying examinations.

The Royal College of Psychiatrists finally emerged from the RMPA but it had been a difficult birth. APIT was threatening to boycott both the examination and the College. Much ill feeling had been engendered in this three-year period and there was considerable anxiety about how the college would function and whether it would be able to differentiate itself from the RMPA. The thesis put forward by the RMPA had been answered by an antithesis put forward by academic and junior psychiatrists in training. This led to a Hegelian synthesis which included the outcomes of much thought and argument. The next chapter shows the differences between the College and the RMPA.

Further reading

Howells, J. G. (1973) The Society of Clinical Psychiatrists. *Bulletin of the Royal College of Psychiatrists*, 6–7.
Howells, J. G. (1991) Re-establishment of the Royal College of Psychiatrists. In *150 Years of British Psychiatry*, Vol. 2 (1841–1991) (eds. G. E. Berrios & H. Freeman). pp. 117–134. Gaskell.

---

13   A Speechless College (1971) *Lancet*, **298**, 914.

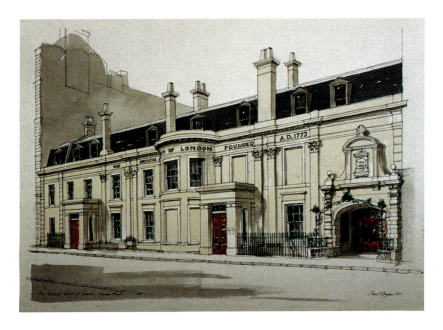

Plate 1 Lettsom House

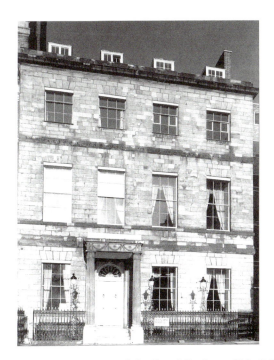

Plate 2 Chandos House, courtesy of the Royal Society of Medicine (from *The History of the Royal Society of Medicine*, by Penelope Hunting (2002))

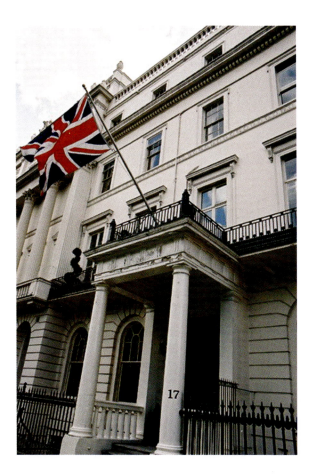

Plate 3   17 Belgrave Square

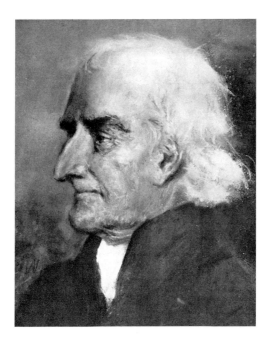

Plate 4 William Tuke

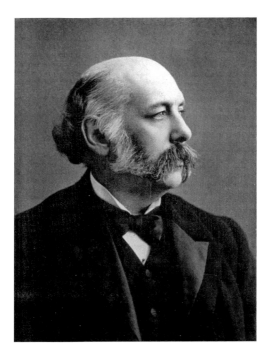

Plate 5 Forbes Winslow

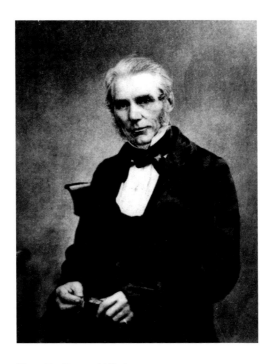

Plate 6   Samuel Hitch

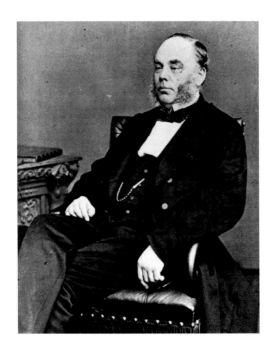

Plate 7   Robert Gardiner Hill

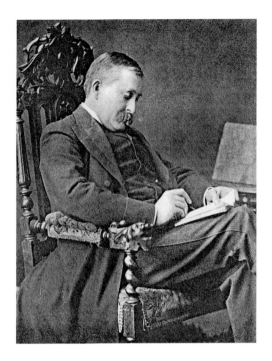

Plate 8 Conolly Norman

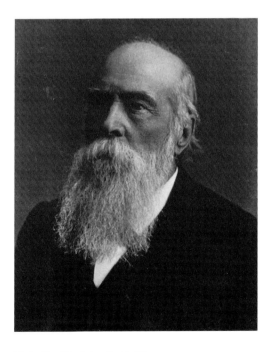

Plate 9 Sir John Bucknill

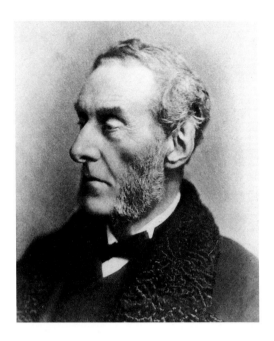

Plate 10 7th Earl of Shaftesbury

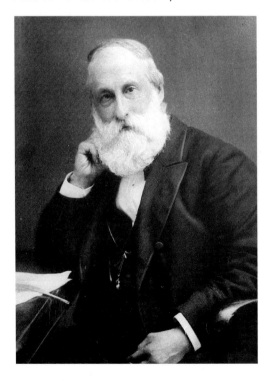

Plate 11 Daniel Hack Tuke

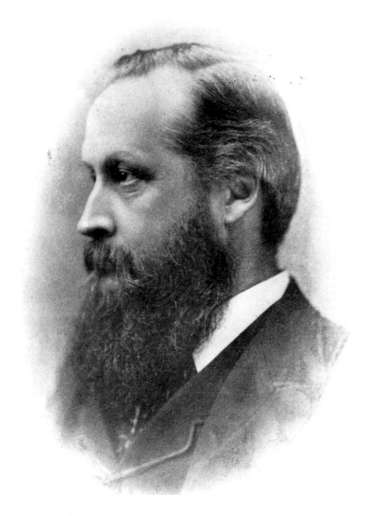

Plate 12 Henry Maudsley

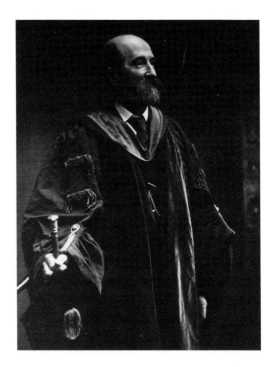

Plate 13 T.S. Clouston

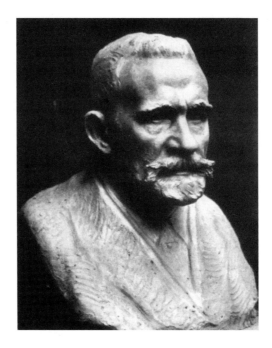

Plate 14 Emil Kraepelin

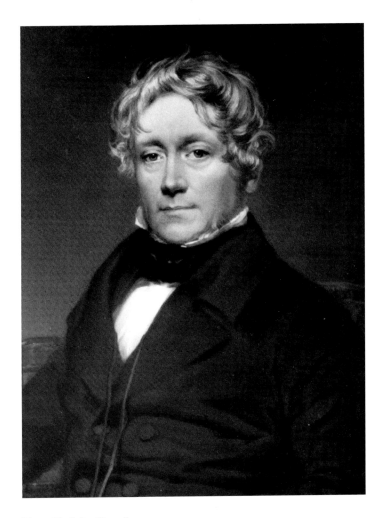

Plate 15 John Conolly

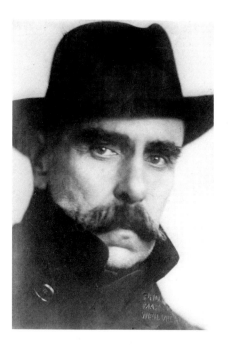

Plate 16 Wagner von Jauregg

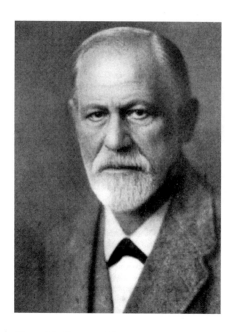

Plate 17 Sigmund Freud

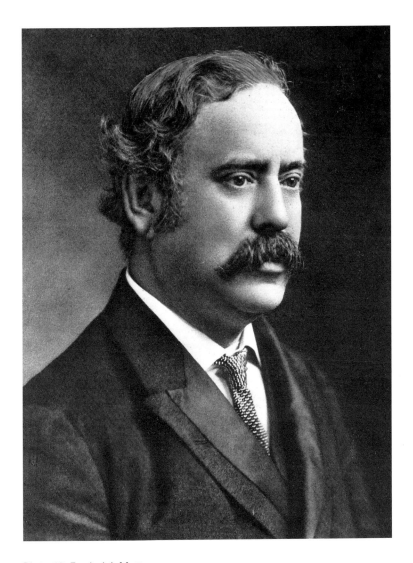

Plate 18 Frederick Mott

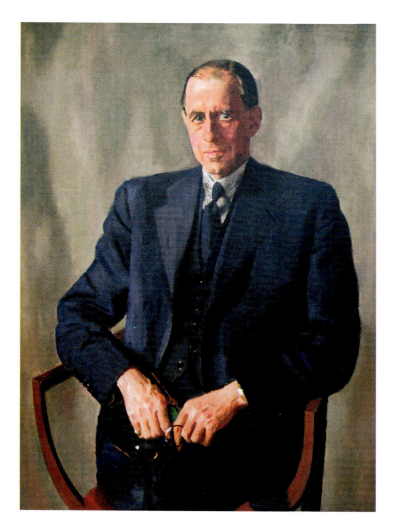

Plate 19 Edward Mapother

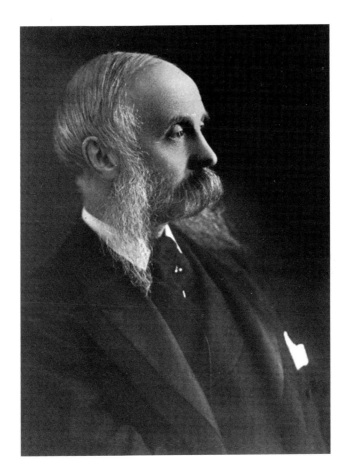

Plate 20 Sir James Chrichton Browne

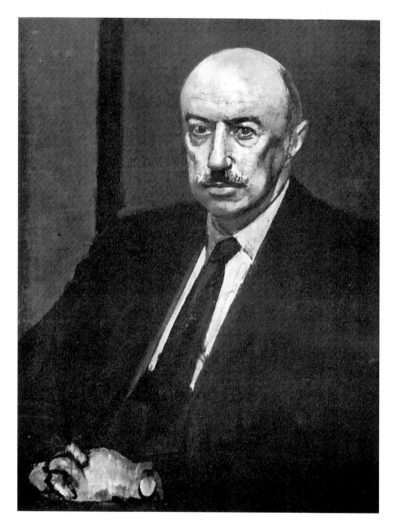

Plate 21 Aubrey Lewis

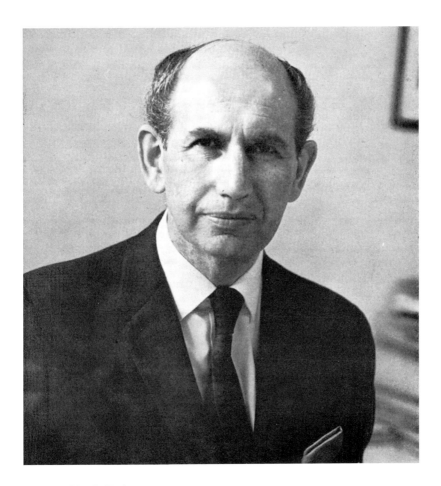

Plate 22 Martin Roth

The Royal College of Psychiatrists 1972–2005

The establishment of the College marked the coming of age of a body that had started in 1841 with 46 members, progressed through its various stages of development, gaining in expertise and influence, and by 1971, had become an established organisation with a membership of almost 4000. The transition from association to college was a time of considerable change in terms of membership entry criteria and election of officers. The first college president brought a period of calm following the turbulence described in Chapter 6. The Association of Psychiatrists in Training provided a vocal body of junior doctors who were prepared to challenge their senior colleagues and who were active in the College's early years. Since then, the College has stabilised and developed to provide in a constructive way what Samuel Hitch and others had envisaged almost 200 years ago. The aims laid down in the College's Charter – teaching, research and public education – have been considerably furthered against a background of steadily diminishing resources for psychiatry.

A Royal College of Psychiatrists was first mentioned in the minutes of the RMPA Council meeting held on 6 July 1948, but it took 24 years to bring the idea to fruition, with opposition both from within and from without. The transition was much more than a change of name. The RMPA Constitution had to be altered considerably to satisfy the Privy Council and ensure that the College would be in a position to accept the challenges of providing ongoing education for psychiatrists in training. This involved the development and inspection of training schemes and an entry examination; the College was not going to be another Association that anyone could join. A second, and crucial, change was the introduction of elections for College officers and Council by postal ballot of the whole membership, rather than by the small number of those who attended meetings regularly. In addition, a body of junior doctors critical of the whole endeavour emerged. Their concern was that the creation of the College would simply involve the introduction of an expensive and compulsory new system of examinations for membership without any other real benefits.

Presidential election and inaugural meeting

Changes came about rapidly. As soon as the College received its Charter elections were held for president, officers and Council. Two-thirds of

Council members and College officers were newly elected and the rest remained from the RMPA. The key change was the election of the first president. The RMPA Council in the transition phase had put forward two names to stand for election: Dr William Sargant, the academic registrar and acting dean, and Dr A. B. Monro, the secretary and acting registrar. Dr J. G. Howells, a member of the Privy Council Committee and one of the leading advocates of the change to collegiate status had also been proposed by 12 RMPA members. The junior doctors, whose actions had led to the success of the Petition Committee, most of whom had become members of the APIT, were not happy with this limited choice. Under the new constitution, it was possible to put forward a further name if proposed by 12 members of the Association who were not Council members and they decided to do so. Professor Martin Roth from Newcastle was approached to stand but would not commit himself until the last day for nominations when he was finally persuaded to allow his name to go forward. This was fortunate as he had the ideal clinical, academic and research experience. He was knighted in 1972.

In the subsequent election, Professor Roth received 578 votes, Dr Sargant 357, Dr Monro 351 and Dr Howells 329. Professor Roth was, therefore, declared president. Dr Sargant, upset that he had not been elected, resigned from his post as Registrar and Professors Bill Trethowan and John Hinton were appointed acting deans until the later election of Professor Kenneth Rawnsley. The College was very fortunate to have elected Martin Roth. Will Sargant was a charismatic individual who had an uncritical view of, and tended to overvalue, some physical treatments, Ben Monro was a mental hospital superintendent and John Howells was the Pied Piper who had led the members into voting for a College. None of the three could have dealt as successfully with the many problems the new College now faced. The months between the granting of the Charter and the formal inauguration of the College had been darkened by the acrimonious dispute with able, talented and articulate younger psychiatrists who considered that their senior colleagues were acting with complacency and self-interest. The College, however, was committed under its Charter to establish a membership examination in psychiatry as soon as possible and a threatened boycott by the junior doctors caused considerable apprehension. A protest of some kind was expected at the inaugural meeting but the first president was determined to reconcile the warring factions. After his induction, Professor Roth gave the Maudsley Lecture (his Charter address), in which he laid out some of the changes that were now required.[1]

'The primary responsibility of the College is the maintenance of standards of professional practice, the upgrading of postgraduate education and the accreditation of hospitals and training programmes. But the provision of

---

1   Roth, M. (1972) The Royal College of Psychiatrists: our immediate tasks and aims. *British Journal of Psychiatry*, **120**, 359–366.

consultants and teachers of psychiatry on a scale that makes it possible to give education high priority and to put psychiatrists into training in numbers adequate to meet realistic estimates of future need, to urge that new buildings be provided and that resources be dedicated to community care, without neglecting the efforts needed to advance the subject by scientific work – all these are inseparable from the quest for higher professional standards. A Royal College could probably get along for a while by confining itself exclusively to matters of immediate practical concern, health administration and education. But it would assuredly die of stagnation if it failed to dedicate some of its energies to fostering the advance of knowledge.

It is not, I think, inappropriate to raise these issues on the present occasion, because it is by pressing forward with scientific endeavour on a wide front and by enlisting the dedicated efforts of bold, gifted and enterprising men at the right time, that disciplines can hope to bring about those salutary advances which have so often transformed whole subjects within a short time. I believe a number of these conditions are satisfied and that a Royal College has an important role in shaping events towards such a general forward movement ... The widespread and growing public concern and involvement with the problems of mental health reflects, among other things, a general appreciation that important advances in the relief of mental suffering would confer immeasurable benefits without damaging side-effects.

The College will be expected to act as a consultative body on "matters of public and professional interest concerning psychiatry and the treatment of mental disorders" (The Charter, 1971). Its views will be sought on the future of the mental hospitals and institutions for the mentally subnormal; on the problem entailed in mounting realistic programmes of community care, without inflicting unfair burdens on families in which spare pairs of female hands are fast vanishing. It will have to consider the changes in perspective, clinical practice and administration that will be demanded as the centre of gravity of the psychiatric team moves to the ambit of the general hospital. With the advent of the College there will be a general desire to give new momentum to such activities by developing working groups of experts, prepared to submit counsel to those with the main responsibility for planning, in which the best that psychiatry can offer in scientific knowledge and practical sense are blended. Psychiatrists are also becoming involved to an increasing extent in problems with even wider social connotations such as drug dependence, alcoholism, crime and violence.

It would be wrong for me to proceed in apparent insensibility of disputes that have divided our College during recent months. Birth-pangs and growing pains were only to be expected but these can often be mitigated by prompt and appropriate action, and there are certain issues which should be squarely faced. There is, moreover, as in other fields, something of a generation gap in views about how things should be done; and the manner in which psychiatrists deal with dissent and disharmony will rightly be judged by the highest standards. Wisdom, empathy and dispassionate decision-making and appreciation of the undercurrents of feeling that often reinforce dissension will be looked for. Such expectations should not be directed towards one side alone ...

I should be evading a duty if I failed to comment on the problem of examinations ... Certain accusations are unfair. We are accused of having slavishly followed in the wake of other bodies which are not appropriate models for a Royal College of Psychiatrists. It is not true that this College, and the Association which preceded it, has concerned itself with examinations without endeavouring to improve education ... I believe there is general agreement that these efforts must be intensified in an attempt to upgrade training programmes and facilities, particularly at peripheral centres. We were irrevocably committed to initiating examinations at the earliest possible date after the granting of the Charter. But as soon as this transitional period is over, there can and will be the most wide-ranging debate about the means that should be adopted to upgrade training. There will also be consultation with the best available psychiatric and educational opinion at all levels of age and seniority as to the fairest and most reliable methods by which the results of training and study may be assessed. Some assessment there has to be and there is no simple and straightforward solution for this. I have always recognised that this must be developed in a manner that engenders a feeling of security among those whom we receive into our field of work, and a mutually rewarding, happy relationship between teachers and the trained. The problem of arriving at a valid and equitable method of assessing competence in a profession is a difficult one. All simple formulae are naive.'

This masterly address did much to defuse the anxieties felt by many junior doctors. Professor Roth ended by comparing the College's proposed examination with that of the competitive examination for posts in the government service of Imperial China a millennium earlier, reassuring that it was not the College's intention to proceed down that road. In an effort to calm anxieties surrounding this issue, he described the ordeal for some 10 000 to 12 000 Chinese candidates over a number of days; at the end some of them were so deranged by stress that they handed in blank paper and copies of the last will. Even the grand examiner himself became unhinged, tearing up the papers handed in and biting and kicking those who approached him till he was finally secured and bound hand and foot to his chair. By now the audience were laughing – the air had been cleared and tension diffused.

Immediately after the Maudsley Lecture, there was an open discussion in which grievances were aired and concessions made regarding exemptions from examination fees. By the end of the day, decisions had been taken and assurances given by the new president. These included the announcement that a Review Committee of five Fellows would independently examine unsuccessful applications for exemption from the membership examination. An anomalous situation had arisen by which those elected to Foundation Membership were to pay a smaller fee on election than those who were to be admitted by examination. It was agreed to explore ways of rectifying this situation that would not contravene the relevant clauses and bye-laws of the Charter. A presidential letter invited foundation fellows and members to pay a sum equivalent to the examination fee in addition to the initial subscription payment.

Membership

Membership of the RMPA had been open to any medically qualified person subject to election and payment of a subscription, whereas full membership of the existing medical Royal Colleges was in general acquired on the basis of a qualifying examination. In the discussions leading up to the foundation of the College, it had been agreed that any psychiatrist of consultant or equivalent status would be entitled to Foundation Membership and those who had over 12 years of service as a consultant would be eligible for Foundation Fellowship. There were still a large number of psychiatrists who had both taken a DPM examination and had been members of the RMPA. These would all automatically become Affiliates of the College but were still subject to the entry examination. This was a transitional category of membership that diminished quickly as those involved took the new Member of the Royal College of Psychiatrists (MRCPsych) exam but it was nonetheless a huge issue at the time and of great concern to junior doctors. The concerns of those who were completing or had completed their training but had not yet been appointed to a consultant post and thus had to take the examination were taken into account. They were granted very substantial exemption from the exam and initially those with a DPM had only to sit a final oral. If they failed that, they were then given the opportunity to sit both an oral and a clinical exam. On failing that, the full membership examination became necessary. One of the effects of these exemptions was that the examination was initially less expensive to run than had been expected and the College made a handsome profit. This caused concern and acrimony among the trainees, and the Council ultimately decided to return the profit to all those who had taken the exam. It was agreed that in future fees for membership examinations would cover costs and nothing more.

Inceptors

A new class of Inceptors was provided for in the College bye-laws approved by the Privy Council. Inceptors were to be the most junior psychiatrists in training who were intending to take the membership examination and become full members. This proved to be a very successful development and there were about 700 Inceptors by the year 2000. The College was the first of the medical Royal Colleges to extend full membership privileges to junior doctors and other Colleges have since followed this example.

Section VI of the College bye-laws read as follows:

'For a period of not more than 10 College years, commencing with the Foundation date, there shall be maintained a register of Inceptors of the College. A qualified medical practitioner may apply to the Court of Electors for registration as an Inceptor, and the Court of Electors may, if it thinks fit, approve his registration as such. An Inceptor shall pay such registration fee as may be prescribed. At the end of each successive year of his registration the status of an

Inceptor shall be reviewed by the Court of Electors which, if it thinks fit, shall renew his registration without further payment by him; provided that, without the special leave of the Court of Electors, no Inceptor may be registered as such for more than five consecutive years, nor may his registration be renewed after he has reached the age of 40 years.'

The category of Inceptor was initially established for a trial period of 10 years. Inceptors were entitled to receive the Journal and to attend scientific meetings but not to vote. If the inceptorship proved to be of value it was open to the College to go back to the Privy Council with a request for the Inceptor class to become a permanent part of its constitution. If it was not a success, the register would close automatically at the end of the trial period or earlier by resolution of a general meeting of the College. The register was opened and there was a steady increase in the number of those joining. In practice, the class of Inceptors in the College proved to be successful and after five years the Privy Council were again approached with a request that the 10-year clause be deleted, making Inceptors a permanent class of the College members.

The Association of Psychiatrists in Training (APIT)

In the first four years after the College was established, the APIT played a major role in the debates and discussion about the way it should develop and function, especially with regard to the membership examination. Trainees from England, Scotland, Wales and Northern Ireland met in Manchester in October 1971 for the first annual College general meeting. The aims set out at the meeting were to:

- represent psychiatric trainees in all matters affecting their interests;
- provide a forum for discussion and action on common problems that trainees in psychiatry may have as a result of the foundation of the Royal College of Psychiatrists;
- act as a pressure group to hasten the establishment and maintenance of adequate training programmes throughout the British Isles and to encourage direct feedback from trainees about such programmes;
- foster meetings and exchanges among trainees and to counter differentials that exist between central and peripheral training hospitals in quality of training facilities.

In the first year of the College, the APIT was extremely active. A regular newsletter – *APIT News* – was published and open forums were arranged with debates on controversial issues in and around psychiatry. These were usually timed to coincide with quarterly College meetings. The APIT also organised twice yearly examination workshops. These concentrated on examination techniques rather than factual knowledge and were held about six weeks before the membership examinations. The APIT had a small executive committee that met regularly and elected a number of regional representatives who were in touch with grass-roots opinion in each psychiatric hospital and had a duty to convey concerns to the executive. This ensured that the APIT was not dominated by those in teaching centres and was representative of junior doctors as a whole.

The issue of trainee representation at every level of the College was raised soon after the inaugural meeting, when it was agreed that there should be a trainee with observer status on all committees. A committee of trainees would become a subcommittee of the Education Committee, to which each region, division and specialty would elect two trainees (one pre and one post membership) and allocate representatives to the other College committees. This eventually became the Collegiate Trainees' Committee. Opposition to the membership examination soon ceased to become a central issue and although the APIT continued to oppose the College over various issues, the relationship became cordial and productive. In the early days, membership slowly grew for a few years to over 5000, but after the development of the Collegiate Trainees' Committee, the need for the APIT gradually diminished and after 10 years the organisation considered that its aims had been achieved and decided to suspend its activities indefinitely.

Collegiate Trainees' Committee

The Collegiate Trainees' Committee (CTC) was a special committee of Council, formed of representatives of senior trainees (a senior trainee is a member with less than four years since election as such) and inceptors (who have not yet passed the membership examination). Its remit was to advise the Council on all matters affecting training and trainees and to represent the interests of trainees within the College and maintain and improve the quality of postgraduate psychiatric training. The CTC was represented on most of the College's committees, including Council (on which the chairman, vice-chairman and honorary secretary were members), and the Executive and Finance Committee (of which the chairman was a member).

Affiliates

In 1994 a new grade of Affiliate was created, specifically to include in the College those who were no longer in training and who did not have the MRCPsych – normally those with what were then referred to as non-consultant career grades. Those who were already affiliates of the College were re-designated Foundation Affiliates. In 2000 a working group was established with the sole aim of taking forward the needs and aspirations of affiliates; a Council Report was produced, which listed a number of recommendations designed not only to help to raise the profile of this long-neglected group of psychiatrists, but also to play a significant role in reviewing the crucial part affiliates play in the everyday running of the National Health Service. They are now represented on most College committees, including Council.

Accreditation and training

The Association of University Teachers of Psychiatry (AUTP) were worried about the College remit to inspect and approve training posts and suggested a committee with the College, leading to the Joint Committee on Higher Psychiatric Training (1971). This consisted of the president, dean and registrar of the College, six members nominated by the College and six by the Association of University Teachers of Psychiatry. Later a representative of the Republic of Ireland and a trainee were added. Its remit was to inspect senior registrar posts. Specialist advisory subcommittees for each of the sub-specialties within psychiatry had been established and were beginning a programme of visits of inspection for recognition of posts. It was agreed that responsibility for the accreditation of training schemes for general professional training as well as the membership examination would remain with the College. The College Dean, Professor Kenneth Rawnsley, (1972–1977), believed that the accreditation exercise was probably more important to the College than the membership examination because it could directly influence the training of psychiatrists in the future. It was intended to be a constructive exercise, spreading information, giving advice and collecting data from all over the country and ensuring adequate standards of training.

At the time of the transition from the RMPA to the College, consideration had been given to standards of training, partly because of concerns expressed by junior doctors and partly because of the decision to accredit suitable training centres. It had been suggested that all the London teaching hospitals should be given full approval automatically but it was decided that all teaching and other hospitals should be dealt with in the same way. This was fortunate as there were many deficiencies in the teaching hospitals and many of them could only be provisionally accredited till their standards had improved.

In the final days the RMPA had circulated a questionnaire to all psychiatric hospitals and units that wished to provide general professional training for the membership examination on the basis of which they would be approved for periods of up to three years. The limitations of the self-administered questionnaire were recognised by Dean Kenneth Rawnsley who felt strongly that visits to units should be carried out. Thus, a preliminary list of accredited hospitals was drawn up and circulated in May 1973. It provided for general classification into two groups:

- hospitals recognised for a full course of training towards the MRCPsych
- hospitals recognised with some limitations in the range of facilities available.

The dean, Professor Ramsey, with Professor Desmond Pond and Dr D. H. Clark made pilot visits to four hospitals looking at both the quality and quantity of teaching and training. Their visits revealed discrepancies between the reality and the paper accreditation exercise as assessed by the hospitals themselves. Some hospitals did not claim to give a complete training and could not, therefore, be accredited as offering such but none the less they were doing a useful job in difficult circumstances. Some, on the other hand, which had seemed on paper to provide full facilities, had totally inadequate organisation and expertise. An accreditation system to take account of both of these possibilities was needed.

Dean Rawnsley set up the system which, with some modifications, was in use for the next 25 years. Each region provided a team of three, led by a convener who went on all visits, to inspect all units in another region and report back to the Dean and the other regional conveners in a meeting of the Central Committee. Their recommendations then went to the College Court of Electors. To start with there were no trainees on such visits, but it soon became virtually mandatory to have a senior (post MRCPsych) trainee as part of the team.

The accreditation exercise was intended to be a two-way process of exchange of information, ideas and views about the best ways of promoting training in various settings. Above all it provided for the first time, through the sanction of possible non-approval, a powerful stimulus to health authorities, trainers and trainees to generate the resources and to organise these into a programme of training in both the theoretical and practical fields. Direct visits were essential for the appraisal of a training programme. The most important evidence was derived from interviews with the trainees themselves, which shed light on the degree of seriousness with which a programme of lectures, seminars, journal clubs and case conferences was actually being implemented by trainers and pursued by trainees. There were other significant benefits as well – the crucial ingredient of supervised clinical experience in a variety of contexts could be assessed; the morale and motivation of staff could be judged against the backcloth of available resources (especially the proportion of medical staff to population); and the time made available for training and study could be checked.

The visiting arrangements were based on the ten divisions of the College covering the whole of the British Isles together with the Channel Islands and military psychiatric units in West Germany. No hospital was visited by a panel from its own regional division. A convener for each division was appointed by consultation between divisions and the Court of Electors. The convener had a panel of colleagues nominated by the division from which he recruited two members to accompany him on each visit. These could include trainees who had obtained the MRCPsych. One benefit of the exercise was the large number of members involved, which brought the importance of training to the top of the College agenda. To minimise variation in criteria used and in the expectations of those being appraised, the convener of each division was present at every primary visit and control of the standards was effectively exercised by the Central Approval Panel comprising the ten conveners and the dean. The Panel received and considered all reports on visits and recommended an appropriate category to the Court of Electors:

- A – approval
- AS – limited approval
- P – provisional approval
- PS – provisional limited approval
- U – not approved

The visits began in January 1974 and the first cycle was virtually completed by January 1977. Hospitals that had been placed in categories P or PS were reassessed about a year after the primary visit.

Over the next five years about half the psychiatric centres in the country were visited. Although the emerging reports were candid and realistic, they were fair and constructive and where criticisms were made they had received serious and responsible consideration. Health authorities had in most cases taken note of the recommendations and in many cases a prompt and practical response was elicited. This was the start of a move to institute proper training schemes in each region with mandatory training in different areas of psychiatry leading to a two-stage examination to be followed by higher specialist training. It was a far cry from the days when some junior psychiatrists were ostensibly trained but did no more than act as a pair of hands for the consultant psychiatrist – the type of training that used to be described as 'sitting by Nellie'. The approval exercises both of new senior registrar posts and of basic training posts at senior house officer and registrar level continued to bring about changes. Many posts, particularly isolated ones, were given only limited approval for a defined period of time and there was a steady move towards larger regional training schemes with rotations between central teaching hospitals and peripheral hospitals. As the approval visits began, training programmes had been improving and rotations were slowly being built up, offering wider experience for junior doctors and more effective teaching opportunities for consultants.

Doctors involved in the inspections also learned much. It emerged that those from the south who had visited northern hospitals were positively impressed with the general standard of decoration of psychiatric hospitals there, which they found perceptibly superior to those in the south. The College's trainees in the north, especially those around major teaching centres there, were on the whole as good as or better than those in most psychiatric hospitals in the south. There was a general dissemination of ideas from the various rotating members on visiting teams. The Central Approval Panel consisted of all the divisional conveners and consensus views were derived from the opinions of members, who would also have local information, thus involving virtually the entire College. In this way, with the dean's guidance, the Panel came to the agreement as to what types of training activities and clinical experience should be encouraged and how much should be expected of individual hospitals, despite quite widely differing circumstances. Not surprisingly, the main information about the training available came from junior doctors, from whom it was possible to verify whether a trainee had ever actually seen a patient with, for example, severe learning disability and whether there were in reality regular case conferences. When a major deficiency in the teaching of a particular senior doctor came to light, the situation was dealt with as tactfully as possible. A number of hospitals were found to be unaware of the considerable length of time off recommended by the Department of Health and Social Security for the education of junior doctors. Sometimes there was no MRCPsych course within a reasonable travelling distance for day-release education or the library and other postgraduate facilities were poor. The trainee rotation was often underdeveloped, so that junior doctors spent too long in one clinical setting.

In five years the College had visited all hospitals at least once and some were visited two, three and more times. There was also a change in that trainees began to be taken on for a three-year training period rather than for a short time in a single post. This was often achieved by pooling the salaries of the trainees and paying them as senior house officers for one or two years and as registrars for the final year. As the College and medicine as a whole developed over the years, postgraduate education has continued to expand. All doctors have had to engage in continuing professional development and must expect to be assessed on their level of competence throughout their professional career. The medical profession through the Colleges, the academy, postgraduate deans, the General Medical Council and the government are all involved. The College thus has a continuing involvement in inspection of training posts and training programmes and for the education, assessment and revalidation of psychiatrists.

The College and the Institute of Psychiatry

The relationship between the College and the Institute of Psychiatry in these early days was interesting. The latter had been dubious about the ability of an organisation they had expected to be run by asylum superintendents to achieve much. No one on the staff there had been willing to stand for election as first president. However, it was following the uprising by junior staff at the Maudsley (described in the previous chapter) that a Council (two-thirds of whom were new) had been elected. Also, the new president, dean and sub-dean had all been in training at the Maudsley earlier, and lastly, the changes introduced by the College were influenced by some of the ideas and practices started by Edward Mapother and Aubrey Lewis.

Postgraduate medical education

The Postgraduate Medical Education and Training Board (PMETB) was established by the General and Specialist Medical Practice (Education and Qualifications) Order, approved by Parliament on 4 April 2003, 'to develop a single, unifying framework for postgraduate medical education (PGME) and training across the UK.' The Board's remit covers basic and higher specialist training but does not cover undergraduate medical education, nor that of pre-registration doctors, which remains the responsibility of the General Medical Council and universities.

The PMETB is responsible for:

- establishing and raising standards and quality in postgraduate medical education and training;
- providing arrangements to ensure this quality is maintained;
- improving supervision of training;
- providing managed structures and processes to ensure all interests are represented in postgraduate medical education;
- regulating specialist and general training.

Specific responsibilities include:

- approval of postgraduate medical education and training programmes and courses;
- accreditation of postgraduate education and training institutions and trainers;
- quality assurance of the postgraduate medical education and training system;
- ensuring that assessments and examinations undertaken as part of training are reliable and fair;
- issuing certificates to doctors meeting the standards it sets for successful completion of training;
- assessing the equivalence of the qualifications, training and experience of doctors seeking a statement of eligibility to apply for entry to the specialist or general practice registers of the General Medical Council.

Despite this major change the College remains heavily involved with postgraduate deans in the organisation and inspection of training programmes in all regions in the UK, and Ireland.

Further College activities

The College has been much more proactive than the RMPA. It became the source of advice to the government on all matters relating to mental health, the role previously performed by the Royal College of Physicians. It also became one of the constituent members of the Conference of Royal Colleges and Faculties of England and Wales. The need for such an organisation had been felt for a considerable time and its work proved to be of importance for the future of British medicine.

Medical audit

There had been a plethora of inquiries that had highlighted a number of serious deficiencies in resources, management, clinical policies and skills in hospitals for the mentally ill and those with learning disabilities. The College set up a special committee on medical audit and one of its first tasks was to investigate the suicides occurring in psychiatric hospitals or units or committed by patients recently discharged. The College also mounted a national inquiry into the use and practice of electroconvulsive therapy (ECT) under the direction of Dr John Pippard, which too was construed as an audit into resources, utilisation and techniques. Dr Pippard found that across the country there were marked differences in the way this treatment was being delivered. It was mostly carried out by inadequately trained junior doctors, with little consultant supervision and much of the equipment in use obsolescent. These findings led to the College issuing guidelines and beginning to set standards, but the first follow-up visits by Dr Pippard showed little improvement. Subsequent checks, however, demonstrated that members of the College were providing better supervision and more adequate training of those learning the proper techniques to be using ETC as well as using up-to-date equipment. Over the years, there was a subsequent decrease in the use of ECT, as many patients did not like the treatment, there was a better awareness of possible adverse effects on memory, and antidepressant drugs came to be used more widely.

Care in the community

With the closure of most of the old large mental hospitals by the end of the 20th century, the focus in recent years has been on care in the community. This can be good rhetoric but the reality can be less than satisfactory. It became more difficult to find hospital places for the chronically mentally ill, many of whom are kept in prisons with no access to appropriate services. The College has voiced much concern about this and about the level of undiagnosed and untreated mental illness that it masks. Successive inspectors of prisons have made these criticisms even more cogently but the situation continues. Although patients who would previously have been in mental hospitals are in general happier to be treated in the community, there remain unsolved problems, at their worst in large cities. Those with mental illness can be neglected and not receive the treatment they deserve. When the NHS was founded, 50% of its budget went to mental health services in the costs of asylums; in 2000 only about 10% of the budget was available for this purpose, hence there is a serious shortage of resources.

A heavy burden is placed on the relatives and carers of those with mental illness or severe learning disabilities. Carer organisations find that unsupported and untrained carers may spend 50 hours a week looking after patients: 86% of them live with the person they look after; 50% of them cannot work and consequently have financial difficulties. There is a grave shortage of acute mental health beds in large cities, which leads to the premature discharge of patients, with occasional catastrophic results. Many of the mentally ill have remained untreated in prison because of the difficulty of finding places for them in hospital units. Mentally ill patients can be neglected, find themselves in gaol, or be cared for by relatives to a much greater extent than was the case when there were more asylums. The College now has a joint committee with relatives and carers to try to provide greater support.

Furthering public education

The College has taken an interest in the prevention of mental illness in terms of both education of the dangers of substance abuse and the links between drug use and excessive alcohol consumption and mental illness. It has endeavoured to follow the precepts in its Charter to 'further public education in the science and practice of Psychiatry'. It launched a 'Defeat Depression' campaign, in partnership with patient organisations, patients and their carers, to increase awareness of this condition and encourage better diagnosis, treatment and acceptance. It has also worked to reduce the stigma of mental illness with a four-year campaign which it supported financially. Research into the effects of this campaign suggested that the public had slightly modified their negativistic views of mental illnesses and patients, although it was unclear whether the campaign had brought this about or whether change was occurring over time for other reasons. There was a book and a website produced as part of the campaign, with relevant information. The College has also tried, in its third major campaign, to reach out to patients and carers as the groups that bear the brunt of all the adverse effects of mental illness.

When the proposal for the Royal College of Psychiatrists first arose, little thought had been given to what this would entail and precisely what role it should play. When it came into being in 1971, most of the officers and Council changed and were subject to intense scrutiny and debate with the membership. Membership examinations were introduced and accreditation and training came to the top of the agenda. It was a period of change and turbulence. At the same time, so-called 'improvements' in the health service leached money from psychiatric resources to shore up other initiatives such as shortening surgical waiting lists. In the years since 1971, the College has expanded in terms of training, research and publishing. Through sensitive leadership, open consultation and compromise, the College has evolved into an effective force for better psychiatric medicine in the 21st century. Much, however, still remains to be done.

CHAPTER 8

Treasurers and finances of the College and its antecedents 1841–2001[1]

The financial state of the Royal College of Psychiatrists and its antecedents, and the concerns, views and activities of the treasurers can be studied through annual accounts and reports, which reveal continuities and differences over the years. Over the 160-year period there were twelve treasurers, who have not been much written about previously; their characters and role are intertwined.[1]

The accounts of the Association of Medical Officers of Asylums and Hospitals for the Insane were first presented in 1851, and are recorded in the handwritten minute book in the College archives. Later the accounts and comments of the treasurer are printed as part of the reports of the annual general meetings in the *Asylum Journal* and its successors. The accounts for 1970 are missing, although the meeting note refers to their having been handed out, and they have been reconstructed from reference to them in 1971. In order not to befuddle the readers with too much detail, and to make comparisons possible, I have examined the accounts at 10 year intervals.

Taverns and subsidies (1841–1871)

The accounts presented in 1851[2] cover the period from 1841 to 1851 and are shown in simplified form in Table 8.1. Formal subscriptions of five shillings each in 1851 were received from 20 members, and the treasurer was evidently out of pocket by seventeen shillings and eightpence. Accounts became more complex later, but similarities of pattern remain, though a 'tavern' is likely to be disguised as a meeting expense.

The first treasurer was Samuel Hitch, resident physician at Gloucester General Lunatic Asylum (1828–1845) and the originator of the letter to 'Medical Gentlemen of Lunatic Asylums' in 1841 which led to the establishment of the Association. He was the secretary and either de facto or appointed treasurer until 1854 when he resigned altogether, possibly in

---

1   This chapter, contributed by Fiona Subotsky, was originally written, in a slightly different form, as a dissertation for the Society of Apothecaries Diploma in the History of Medicine, 2003.

2   RMPA, Minute Book 1, pp. 56–57. College archives.

Table 8.1. The early accounts of the Association (1841–1851). Data presented in pound sterling.

Receipts	1841	1847	1848	1849	1850–1851	Totals
'In hand'		11				11
Subscriptions		1			5	6
Expenditure						
Stationery, postage etc	2	3	2	2	2	11
Printing		2		1	2	5
Tavern					2	2
Surplus/deficit						−1

a huff.[3,4] What happened to him subsequently remains obscure, although he left Gloucester and established a private asylum. A note in the College archives says that 'not a veil but a mackintosh [was drawn] over his later years.'[5]

Samuel Hitch was followed in his post by William Ley, who remained treasurer until 1863. He was the Medical Superintendent of the County Asylum, Littlemore, Oxfordshire, and chairman of the Association in 1848. In 1861, the accounts represented a satisfactory state of affairs. Income was largely from subscriptions received (£233) and from the sale of the Journal (£69). Expenditure was on the Journal and printing (£111), annual and other meetings, and sundries and 'other' (£6); the within-year surplus was £29 and the overall balance was over £75.[6] Ley resigned in 1863,[7] apparently because of ill-health, and a vote of thanks to him was proposed for his 'very energetic and very effectual' services.

In Ley's obituary[8] there is no remark on his treasurership but it is noted that it was when he presided over the meeting at Oxford in 1848 that the establishment of a journal was decided upon. His key role in initiating and

---

3   Tuke, D. H. (1879) *Historical Sketch of the Association. General Index to the First Twenty-Four Volumes of the Journal of Mental Science*, pp. iii–viii.

4   Wood, T. O. (1896) The early history of the Medico–Psychological Association. *JMS*, **42**, 241–260.

5   Anonymous note dated 1963. *The Descendants of John Hitch*. College archives: biographical notes.

6   Official Report. Association of Medical Officers of Asylums etc. (1861) *JMS*, **7**, 309–331.

7   Annual Meeting (1863) *JMS*, **9**, 421–424.

8   Obituary of William Ley (1869) *JMS*, **15**, 166.

supporting the *Asylum Journal* under the editorship of John Bucknill is also mentioned by Hack Tuke in 1896 (albeit with a slightly different account of events).[9] It seems clear that the Journal was of crucial significance in maintaining the objectives of the Association in terms of promoting learning and interprofessional communication. Ley was 'a modest unobtrusive man [who] performed with scrupulous diligence his daily work ... regularly attended the annual meetings of the Medico–Psychological Association and took an unwearying interest in its work and success'.[10] His ill-health was thought by himself and others to be related to his clinical work, of which it was said that it was a special feature of his management that the patients were invariably treated with gentleness. He had remarked himself that 'It took more out of a man than any man is justified in giving'.[11]

Emeritus Treasurer

At the 1871 annual meeting[12] a proposal was put forward to open membership (standing at 300) to other interested medical men (specifically not ladies) and others. Henry Maudsley, in the chair, threatened the arrival of Spiritualists and Swedenborgians and the final agreement was for an associate membership category. John Hayball Paul, Treasurer from 1863 to 1894, presented the accounts – while income and expenditure had increased in comparison with 1861, the pattern was similar; the within-year surplus was £25 and the final balance was £84.

In 1881[13] the balance sheet presented by Paul was accepted with something of a relief and he himself received thanks for 'the admirable way in which he had kept [the accounts], and for the handsome balance of £255 which he was able to show at the end of the year.' This sudden enthusiasm perhaps made a change of mood from a preceding uneasy exchange about the Journal – as in fact there was a within-year loss of £28 and so the balance had actually declined from the previous year.

The accounts for 1890–1891 were presented by Hack Tuke as John Paul could not be present.[14] Few members suggested investing some of the balance of £290, considering it 'unbusiness-like to keep so large an amount in cash'. The president, however, was opposed to this as he thought it could jeopardize the College funds, especially that there had been a within-year deficit of £86. A major difficulty was an increase in Journal

---

9   Tuke, D. H. (1879) *Historical Sketch of the Association. General Index to the First Twenty-Four Volumes of the Journal of Mental Science*, pp. iii–viii.

10   Obituary of William Ley (1869) *JMS*, **15**, 166.

11   Mr Ley of Littlemore (1869) *JMS*, **15**, 315–317.

12   Proceedings of the Twenty-Sixth Annual General Meeting of the Medico–Psychological Association (1871) *JMS*, **17**, 438–452.

13   Report of the Thirty-Sixth Annual General Meeting of the Medico–Psychological Association (1881) *JMS*, **27**, 435–440.

14   Medico–Psychological Association of Great Britain and Northern Ireland. Jubilee Year (1891) *JMS*, **37**, 639–645.

costs without a concomitant income – and there was as yet no income from advertisements.

John Hayball Paul was the longest serving treasurer. He had founded Camberwell House Asylum in 1846. After Paul's death, in 1899, Spence remarked in his presidential address that 'the death of Dr Paul severs one of the last links connecting the modern with the old and barbarous method of dealing with the insane.'[15] Paul's obituary noted that, 'In the days now long gone by, when money was scarce and members few, the Treasurer of the Association practically kept the Association going by the generous expenditure of considerable sums which he never mentioned ... A wealthy man who dispensed charity with a liberal hand, he was always a kind, sympathetic friend, considerate and courteous to all, an honourable and upright man in all his dealings.'[16] If Paul actually subsidised the Association as opposed to helping out with the cash flow his popularity is hardly surprising. After he left office he was elected Emeritus Treasurer.

Consolidation of investments and subscriptions (1901–1921)

The treasurer's office was subsequently taken by Herbert Hayes Newington (President 1889, Treasurer 1894–1917). In 1901,[17] he gave details of income and expenditure in a somewhat defensive manner: 'Upon the whole the Association is doing very well; it pays its way with a little over.' On the Journal: 'It is entirely in the hands of the editors, who are men of experience ... [its] sale ... is uncertain, about £200.' On examinations: 'an extra 2s 6d had been charged to each nursing candidate, which goes to the examiners. The miscellaneous account had heavier than usual expenditure on printing ... There is a dividend income of £13 10s 8d; a sum of £336 was collected as a testimonial to Dr Hack Tuke – the interest of that goes to the library account.' On the handbook: '[its] sale ... is very uncertain; it seems to be going on as usual.' There was a considerable increase of advertisements in the Journal. 'The fees for the Psychological Certificate in Medicine are very small indeed; they used to be a very fruitful source of income. Now the cost of examining these gentlemen is a great deal more than the money we get from them.' He added that an additional expense was that, on the occasion of the death of the late Queen, the Association voted an address of condolence to His Majesty which cost ten guineas.

What followed was a heated discussion, prompted by a surplus of only £44, at which some members expressed 'disquiet'. Others rose to the treasurer's defence, saying that he can only save money where there is some.

---

15   Spence, J. B. (1899) Presidential Address. *JMS*, **45**, 637.

16   Obituary: John Hayball Paul (1899) *JMS*, **45**, 430–431.

17   Medico–Psychological Association of Great Britain and Ireland: Annual Meeting (1901) *JMS*, **47**, 836–840.

The members were asked to make an effort, for instance by persuading advertisers to use the Journal.

In fact, in comparison with ten years before, the range and size of receipts (now including advertisements) was increasing and the overall closing balance was a healthy £1223. Decisions had clearly been made to invest some of the surplus after all and these were literally paying dividends. Mention is made of rent to 11 Chandos Street; the Association had begun to lease space there from the Medical Society of London in 1893.[18]

The examinations referred to in the treasurer's report were a notable feature of the accounts for many years – Certificate of Proficiency in Nursing (for asylum nurses, 1891) and Certificate in Psychological Medicine (for doctors, 1885). The sale of the *Handbook for the Instruction of Attendants of the Insane* (1885) also generated income over the years.

Ten years later, in 1911,[19] Newington, still the treasurer, could report generally that the affairs of the Association were in a satisfactory condition. The auditors noted that 114 members were in arrears, and that income from the sale of the handbook had fallen off. 'We cannot conclude without renewing the congratulations which have formed a feature of previous auditors' reports to the Treasurer on the excellent and business-like condition of the accounts and affairs of the Association, and we desire to express the hope that he will for many years be able to continue his great services in this capacity.' Newington, who seemed to have a better grasp than the auditors, and was being more assertive this time, was pleased to have the unpaid subscriptions remarked upon, as they did cause 'unnecessary trouble'. His view on the handbook was that the income for this year was normal, the previous year having been exceptionally high because of a new edition. The closing balance was £2234, the opening balance having been £2086; membership stood at 730.

Herbert Hayes Newington was the medical superintendent of Ticehurst House. His presidential address *Hospital Treatment for Recent and Curable Cases of Insanity*[20] is notable for a mathematical analysis of how many beds would be needed according to an estimate of throughput, which perhaps gives an indication of his systematic approach as treasurer. He was valued both as a treasurer and an active member of the Association – he served on nearly all the committees, and 'rare indeed must have been the occasions when his advice was not followed.'[21] He was also very influential politically in gaining amendments to legislation.

---

18   Harcourt Williams, M. (1999) Royal College of Psychiatrists' archives: the search for accommodation. *Psychiatric Bulletin*; **23**, 761.

19   The Medico–Psychological Association of Great Britain and Ireland (1911) JMS, **57**, 723–729.

20   Newington, H. H. (1889) Presidential Address. *JMS*, **35**, 293–315.

21   The Medico–Psychological Association of Great Britain and Ireland (1913) *JMS*, **59**, 694–696.

After the Great War

In 1921 the membership was reported as 656 and had not yet recovered to the pre-war level.[22] This is reflected in the reduced number of subscriptions in comparison with ten years previously. In the 1920 balance sheet submitted by James Chambers (president 1913–1914, treasurer 1917–1931), the excessive cost of printing the Journal emerged – it was considerably more than members' subscriptions and a committee was appointed to look into the matter. There was a within-year deficit in the revenue account of about £40, but overall the assets had continued to increase in value.

War and change (1931–1971)

Membership stood as 847 in 1931,[23] having by then improved on the pre-war position. While the epithet of 'Royal' has now been attained (in 1926), there are no remarks on this, the novelty having presumably worn off. The Treasurer submitted the revenue account and balance sheet for 1930, and also the financial statement of the Maudsley bequest and of the Gaskell Fund. The Association purchased £800 of 3.5% conversion loan. The accounts show that the subscription income had almost doubled over ten years. There was a within-year revenue account surplus of £587 and a closing balance of £16273, contributed to by increase in value of the investments and the appearance of a Mott memorial fund of £235. The Maudsley bequest, of £2000, had been received in 1918, and was used to fund a lecture. (Henry Maudsley, who was president of the Association in 1871, is primarily remembered today as the founder, with a donation of £30000 to the London County Council, of the then Maudsley Hospital in Denmark Hill.)

In 1931 James Chambers had resigned his post as treasurer, owing to ill-health. He was the medical superintendent of the Priory Roehampton, and in his presidential address *Prevention of the Insanities* recommended segregation of the unfit and 'the necessity for personal effort'.[24] On his death in 1938 the President described him as 'a man [of] fine and dignified appearance … honest purpose and … devoted and conscientious work'.[25] Chamber was 'a modest self-effacing man … trusted by all; regarded with affection by all', but notably, there are no comments in his obituary on his achievements or skills as treasurer, despite the fact that over the course of his tenure the financial position of the Association continued to improve greatly.

---

22   The Medico–Psychological Association of Great Britain and Ireland (1921) Eightieth Annual General Meeting. *JMS*, **67**, 511–517.

23   The Royal Medico–Psychological Association of Great Britain and Ireland (1931). Ninetieth Annual General Meeting. *JMS*, **77**, 862–876.

24   Chambers, J. (1913) The presidential address on the prevention of the insanities. *JMS*, **59**, 549–582.

25   The Royal Medico–Psychological Association. Ninety-Seventh Annual Meeting. Obituary (1938) *JMS*, **84** (suppl., September), 1–2.

Although 1941 was the centenary year, because of wartime conditions it was decided not to regard the meeting that year as a commemorative meeting. The number of members had temporarily reduced somewhat because of the war and relative lack of committee meetings. However, George William Smith (treasurer 1931–1946) reported that the finances of the Association were in good health as was shown by an excess of income over expenditure in all the funds. He had been able to invest £1700 in 2.5% war bonds. The revenue account showed a within-year surplus of £251. From the 1931 level, despite the increase in members, the subscription income had fallen, indicating, presumably, a collection problem.[26]

When George William Smith retired in 1946,[27] the president reminded members that '[he] was responsible among other great services for enlarging the 1920 edition of the Handbook … and the Association remained in a prosperous state owing to his untiring work.' Dr Smith's response sounds rather tired, saying that 'he was getting on in life now and the finances of the Association had not been easy for the past five years. The treasurer received the money, and paid it out and took advantage of gilt-edged investments, and got the praise for it. The subscription list had become complicated because of absence on war service and he had no hesitation in saying that Dr Tennent would take over a very tedious job … He would recommend the Council to strike off those who would not heed the Treasurer's reminders.' Clearly he was still having problems with poor payers. No obituaries have so far been located (Smith died in 1961), perhaps because of missing Supplements, but Smith was recognised in his time and received an OBE. He was made an honorary member of the Association in 1944.

The membership, at 1179 in 1951, had been steadily increasing over the previous five years. A decrease in the number of entries in the Nursing Examinations was noted. Thomas Tennent (treasurer 1947–1962, president 1952) reported a revenue account deficit of £538, which would have been worse had not the examinations made a profit of £99. The previous year the subscription was raised by one guinea, but most of this had been absorbed and further economies were necessary. The main expenditure was in respect of the offices and the publication of the Journal. The net cost of the latter during the year had been £2700; it had been agreed to restrict this to £1750. The increased end-of-year balance was due to a growth in the value of investments.[28]

Ten years on, in 1961, Tennent reported a surplus amounting to £409, compared with £2591 in 1959. The main item of increased expenditure was still the Journal, whose publication in 1960 cost £3742 – various steps were

---

26   The Royal Medico–Psychological Association. Annual Meeting (1941) *JMS*, **87** (Supplement, October), 1–7.

27   The Royal Medico–Psychological Association. One Hundred and Fifth Annual Meeting (1946) *JMS*, **92** (suppl., October), 2.

28   The Royal Medico–Psychological Association. One Hundred and Tenth Annual Meeting (1952) *JMS*, **98** (suppl., October), 1–12.

taken to reduce this. There is no reference to examinations – at this stage the Association had ceased to run the examination for nurses (the last were held in 1951).[29]

Thomas Tennent, a medical superintendent of St Andrew's, Northampton (1938–1962), was 'a dry, laconic, clear-sighted man, firm in his friendships, who spoke his mind plainly but was free from rancour and sentimentality.'[30] He died in office in 1963. That year the credit balance was £47 000, an improvement mainly attributed to the fact that the Journal's financial problems were resolved. This was certainly a key issue, and was to recur.

The first annual meeting of the newly formed Royal College of Psychiatrists was held in November 1971, the incoming president being Martin Roth.[31] An important change relevant to the finances was the introduction of examinations for membership of the College – a qualification related to competence to practise at consultant level. There had been much debate on the 'transitional procedures' governing entitlement to membership of the new College, without passing the examination, and on the details of the new examination itself. The proposed subscription rate for standard membership was for £25 initially and £17 annually. Those who would have to pay considerably more to achieve membership by examination objected to this as unfair, and curiously it was agreed that Foundation Members and Foundation Fellows should make a payment at least equal to that asked of examination candidates. In 1970 the Journal was in deficit by £6907, a state of affairs which worsened the following year. With the main possible sources of income – subscriptions, examinations and publications – in flux, this was obviously a period of great financial uncertainty as well as major change. A sum of money was made available for a feasibility study relating to an appeal for funds for a College building. The appeal was subsequently undertaken, very successfully, and enabled the purchase of the lease of 17 Belgrave Square.

Wilfrid Warren, a consultant child psychiatrist at the Royal Bethlem and Maudsley Hospitals, was treasurer from 1962 to 1979. He was highly praised for his 'supreme ability in handling money matters, not least of all his decision to stand firm on the decision to buy 17 Belgrave Square.'[32] However, Martin Roth's obituary casts a slightly different light: 'Although unflappable, he responded with a combination of grief and panic to potentially ruinous interest rates to which we were pledged under the terms of the huge loan (guaranteed) we were compelled to float in order to purchase Belgrave Square ... Wilfred's equanimity was restored [by] an ingenious and highly

29   The Royal Medico–Psychological Association. One Hundred and Twenty First Annual Meeting (1962) *JMS*, **108** (suppl., January), 1–11.

30   Tennent, T. (1962) *Munk's Roll*, **5**, 408.

31   Royal College of Psychiatrists. Minutes of the First Annual Meeting (1973) *British Journal of Psychiatry*, **121** (News and Notes, June) 3–11.

32   The College. Minutes of the Eighth Annual Meeting (1979) *Bulletin of the Royal College of Psychiatrists*, **3**, 181.

favourable arrangement with an obscure and distant branch of Barclay's Bank.'[33] Warren's successor, Michael Pare, paid tribute to Warren, who 'at a time when the stock market was falling managed not only to maintain, but to increase the College's funds.'[34]

Crisis and recovery (1981–2001)

The 1980s began for the College moderately well, with a revenue surplus of £114 397. Publications made a major contribution to this (mainly from advertisements) with a surplus of over £90 000. Yet the treasurer, Michael Pare (in office 1979–1986), warned that in a period of recession and inflation it would be unwise to be too dependent on the Journal sales, and proposed a rise in the subscription rate and an annual review in the light of inflation. Examinations made a loss of £6564 and the fees were to be raised as a result. On the whole, the College finances were relatively healthy and the accumulation of £783 594 in the General Fund and £618 103 from the Appeal Fund had provided the £1 040 847 spent in acquiring the lease and equipping Belgrave Square. Meanwhile, the College's investment portfolio was £437 350. Pare was concerned that the lease had 53 years to run and it was important to put aside money to buy the lease or alternative accommodation at the end of this time, and proposed that £50 000 should be set aside annually for this.[35] He was right to introduce a note of caution, as office expenses had increased tenfold over ten years and the income stream from investments was major but uncertain.

Charles Michael Bromiley Pare was a consultant at St Bartholomew's Hospital. He was introduced in 1987 as an honorary fellow, by Thomas Bewley, as follows: 'Dr Pare appears to have been able to both increase the value of the College's funds and extend its building without cutting back on normal expenditure,' and somewhat ambiguously, 'wisdom and probity are the qualities required of a Treasurer rather than fiscal ability or numeracy and Dr Pare had the necessary qualities in abundance.'[36] Curiously, Pare's obituaries refer to his research in depression, his authorship of many books, his proficiency at golf and his jovial personality, but not to his role as treasurer.

The 1991 accounts[37] are in a particularly opaque format. William Dalziel Boyd, treasurer 1986–1993, noted that the main source of deficit in the

33   Roth, M. (1991) Obituary: Wilfred Warren. *Psychiatric Bulletin*, **15**, 458–459.
34   The College. Minutes of the Ninth Annual Meeting (1980) *Bulletin of the Royal College of Psychiatrists*, 4, 196.
35   The College. Minutes of the Tenth Annual Meeting (1981) *Bulletin of the Royal College of Psychiatrists*, **5**, 231–239.
36   The Sixteenth Annual Meeting (1987) *Bulletin of the Royal College of Psychiatrists*, **11**, 411–412.
37   Royal College of Psychiatrists (1991) *Eighteenth Annual Report*. Royal College of Psychiatrists.

93

general revenue account was due to an accounting provision for the decline in value of equities of over £35000. Examinations and Public Education Departments were well within budget and Publications showed a healthy surplus. Costs of meetings had increased and had been affected by the reduced financial assistance given to members for travel. Boyd stressed that any extra spending should come from subscriptions, which had to be reviewed every year. However, while the accounts at first glance show a healthily increased closing balance for that year, this includes a large bank loan, the need for which is far from apparent. Subsequently a period of great financial difficulties ensued.

An interview with Bill Boyd was published in 1997.[38] He commented on his time as the College's treasurer that there were 'increasing activities, greater demands, more expectations from the members, more expectations from the public about what pronouncements should come out of Belgrave Square, more involvement in political matters, more involvement with [National Health Service] matters at local level, a need for more staff in the College and therefore a need for more resources, but all this happening in a very exciting way.'

In 2001, the treasurer (myself) noted that as the College's largest source of income was from members' subscriptions it was a cause of satisfaction that the membership had increased to over 10000.[39] However, in 2000 there was a less good climate for investment and for fund-raising, and as a result the surplus was less than for the previous year. Many worthwhile activities and developments were supported, in line with the charitable objectives – especially the Anti-Stigma Campaign (1998–2003). The introduction of tiered subscription rates was proposed for overseas members and for those with reduced incomes for reasons such as taking maternity leave or working part-time. The surplus from the Examinations Department was a cause for discussion with the trainees as to how the College could use this to benefit both the examination system in general and the trainees themselves.

There had been marked changes within the preceding ten years, which a single snapshot cannot fully depict. Israel (Issy) Kolvin had been treasurer from 1993 to 1999. The previous administrative head of finance had left suddenly with the accounts in a state of disarray, and the new head, together with Issy, pulled the finances back into stability with intensive personal efforts and the establishment of a Finance Management Committee, accountable to the Executive and Finance Committee, to oversight the process. Issy also introduced the 'Development Fund' levy on income-generating activities such as conferences to go towards College initiatives and savings towards a building fund.

Issy Kolvin had started his medical career in South Africa, and spent most of his professional life in Newcastle as a highly respected academic in child

38   Tait, D. (1997) Interview: Bill Boyd. *Psychiatric Bulletin*, **21**, 769–774.
39   Royal College of Psychiatrists (2000) *Annual Report and Accounts*. Royal College of Psychiatrists.

psychiatry. In 1990 he became Professor of Child and Family Mental Health at the Royal Free Hospital School of Medicine and the Tavistock Centre, where he continued his studies of evidence bases for treatment. Within the Royal College of Psychiatrists he had been vice president, chairman of the Child and Adolescent Psychiatry Section, and treasurer, and became an Honorary Fellow in 2000. In his nomination for the Fellowship Fiona Caldicott remarked: 'Issy has also shown the importance of (teamwork) throughout his career in all manner of ... settings, and nowhere more effectively than when as fellow Officers we successfully addressed the Royal College of Psychiatrists' mounting financial deficit from 1993 to 1996'.[40]

By 2001, the Royal College of Psychiatrists had over 10 000 members in the UK, Ireland and overseas and was a prosperous organisation able to devote resources to research and public education as well as more immediate member activities. This was not achieved entirely smoothly and certainly there were worries for the treasurers from time to time. However, many, especially in the earlier years, had major managerial responsibilities in still-famous institutions, where they no doubt used and developed financial skills. Themes causing financial anxiety tended to recur: the need for increased membership, and for members to pay their subscriptions; the state of the examinations; the Journal expenditure; the expenses of meetings and administration; the need to pay for premises. Treasurers, as Boyd remarked, have to keep pointing out the need for caution. Psychiatry does not usually generate a large flow of donations, and psychiatrists did not always ensure a surplus on potentially income-generating activities such as publications and examinations. Probably the most importantly helpful financial decisions were to invest some degree of surplus, to aim for advertisements, and to launch an appeal for the purchase of the Belgrave Square building. Of course, the achievement of the 'Royal College' status helped enormously in extending membership, standards and prestige. While James I of England remarked that 'all treasurers if they do good service to their masters must be generally hated', the psychiatrists' treasurers seem, on the whole, to have been appreciated by their fellows.

---

40   Twenty-ninth Annual Meeting (2000) *Psychiatric Bulletin*, **24**, 475.

CHAPTER 9

Development of specialties

Some degree of specialism within psychiatry began to emerge in the 19th century, but the work was continued more fully in the second half of the 20th century. The first special hospitals for the 'criminally insane' were opened in the 1860s, and some psychiatrists in the Association regularly gave evidence to the courts in criminal cases. Separate hospitals called 'idiot colonies' or asylums developed to care for people with severe learning disability. Doctors from all disciplines dealt with disturbed children before child psychiatry developed in England from the child guidance movement and psychoanalysis. Psychotherapy began to be seen as a separate specialty with the development of psychoanalysis and psychoanalytical training institutes in the 20th century. An increasingly ageing population as well as a steady rise in the amount of alcohol consumed and the use of socially prohibited drugs led to the emergence of two further specialties – Old Age Psychiatry and Substance Misuse Psychiatry. There had been little formal training in any of these specialties till after the Second World War, though there had been some such bodies as the Institute of Psychiatry of London University and the Institute of Psychoanalysis that dealt with these issues.

Forensic psychiatry

Forensic psychiatry has a long history. In 1841 (the year the Association was founded) a leading article in the *Lancet* drew attention to 'one of the most difficult questions in jurisprudence or in morals … the difficulty of determining the precise lines of demarcation between the extremes of bad temper, fanaticism and the commencement of actual insanity.'[1]

In 1843 the case of Daniel McNaughten, who attempted to kill the then prime minster, but killed his private secretary instead, led to acquittal with a defence of insanity. In consequence, the McNaughten Rules were formed. They stated that for a successful defence of insanity it must be clearly proved that 'at the time of committing the act the party accused was labouring under such a defect of reason, from disease of the mind, as not to know the nature and quality of the act he was doing, or if he did know it, that he did not know

---

1   Leading article (1843) *Lancet*, 18 March, 903–906.

what he was doing was wrong.'[2] As a result, it became virtually impossible for the law in England to develop or to recognise the concept of diminished responsibility (which was accepted in Scotland in 1867) until the Homicide Act 1957, which then included the possibility of 'irresistible impulse'.

Criminal lunatic asylums were opened in Dublin in 1845 for Ireland and at Broadmoor in 1863 for England. Initially those who worked in these special hospitals were forensic psychiatrists. They were also called in as experts, for example Henry Maudsley and Forbes Winslow, to help the courts decide on responsibility in difficult and serious criminal cases. A forensic psychiatrist was no longer simply a specialist (a 'mad doctor' or an 'alienist') but a doctor who needed to be familiar with the principles of the criminal law, the functioning of its multifarious agencies, the reasoning behind sentences and the reactions of society. Senior psychiatrists also advised the Home Secretary after conviction, especially about capital punishment until it was abolished.

The MPA and the RMPA were regularly concerned with medico–legal issues which frequently surfaced in presidential addresses. These included: issues of wrongful confinement, procedures of certification, the lack of conformity between doctors and lawyers in the legal definition of insanity (particularly in relation to the insanity plea and the boundary between mental illness and criminal responsibility). With the introduction of the Mental Health Act 1959 and Mental Health Act 1960, which allowed detention of a mentally disordered person in hospital and detention with restrictions on discharge, the RMPA began to form a specialist group to discuss these issues and to formulate its policy to Ministers and others. There was no formal Forensic Psychiatry Section in England, although the Scottish Division had one. In 1961 in England and Wales an informal group of senior medical superintendents and deputy superintendents began to meet to discuss forensic psychiatry matters, with membership by invitation. In addition the RMPA Research and Clinical Committee had a subcommittee on forensic psychiatry. On the first general meeting of the Royal College of Psychiatrists it was proposed and agreed that a Forensic Section should be established. The news supplement of the College Journal in April 1973 published the names of the first officers and executive committee of the (then) four specialist sections (i.e. Forensic, Psychotherapy, Mental Subnormality and Child Psychiatry) all elected by ballot.[3]

In 1997, along with the other main sections of the College, the Forensic Section became a Faculty with greater opportunities to develop its activities and oversee training standards. A Mental Health Law Committee took on scrutiny of the legislative issues that affect the mentally ill and an Ethics Committee was established.

---

2   West, D. J. & Walk, A.(eds) (1977) *Daniel McNaughten: His Trial and the Aftermath*, p. 75. Gaskell.
3   News and Notes (1973) April, 2.

Learning disability psychiatry

Difficulty in learning can cause problems with various levels of severity. Those once called 'feeble minded' can learn a certain amount but considerably less than their peers. Those who can learn virtually nothing were once called 'idiots' or 'imbeciles'. The latter often also had physical handicaps and symptoms of brain damage, such as epilepsy. Such people were generally cared for by their families. When this was not possible, for instance because of severe behavioural problems, they might be placed in a workhouse or prison. When asylums were first built some were detained there. A later development was what were called 'idiot colonies' or 'idiot asylums', which eventually became hospitals for the mentally handicapped. With the closure of asylums, people with learning disability are again looked after in the community by their families. They should be helped by services in the community, namely day centres, special schools, training facilities and sheltered workshops. Those with the most severe handicaps (including severe physical disabilities) may need total lifetime care in designated units.

The RMPA had a Mental Deficiency Committee which was the focus for expertise in mental handicap. This paved the way for the formation of a Mental Deficiency Section in 1946 to represent the specialist interest within the RMPA. In 1965 part of a legacy left to the RMPA on the death of Dr R. J. Blake Marsh, first secretary and subsequent chairman of the mental deficiency section, was used to found an annual lecture on a subject connected with mental deficiency. The lecture was to be known by his name and the first such lecture was delivered in 1967. In 1994 the Mental Deficiency Section became the Learning Disability Faculty.[4]

Child psychiatry

Children's behaviour has always created problems for adults and has sometimes indicated mental dysfunction – reactions have varied through the centuries. Behavioural disorders could be seen as moral problems deserving punishment, while failure to learn could lead to a marginal existence as a village fool. Only rarely were childhood mental problems dealt with by doctors. Changes came about for two reasons: concern about educational failure and new psychological ideas about infant and childhood development. In the early part of the 20th century child guidance clinics, sometimes associated with courts, were established and the triumvirate of child psychiatrist, social worker and educational psychologist worked there with children. Paediatricians and psychotherapists were often involved as well. A new discipline of child psychiatry, based on the study of emotional development and epidemiology, slowly emerged, owing to the work of

---

4   Online archive 25*b*. Learning disability.

such outstanding clinician researchers as Michael Rutter. Child psychiatry services are generally now incorporated in Child and Adolescent Mental Health Services (CAMHS).

There are some references in the RMPA Council's early minutes to children (behaviour of delinquents and children in asylums) but these are not very frequent. In the 1930s the RMPA seemed to have become more aware of the needs of children and its representative was appointed to a government committee on mentally defective children. This may have led to the formation of the Child and Adolescent Psychiatry Section. In 1942 the RMPA set up a Child Guidance Subcommittee, renamed the Child Psychiatry Subcommittee in March 1943 and becoming the Child Psychiatry Section in 1946. It was sometimes called the 'children's section' in early minutes and was the Child and Adolescent Psychiatry Section from the early 1980s until 1997 when it became the Faculty of Child and Adolescent Psychiatry.[5]

Psychotherapy

While mesmerism and its successor hypnotism were the most popular psychological treatments of the 19th century, two developments in the last century are the basis of most psychotherapy today: the psychoanalysis of Sigmund Freud and behavioural approaches.

Present-day psychotherapy owes much to Sigmund Freud. He wrote in such a way that his ideas influenced the psychiatric practice much more than his attempts to treat minor nervous disorders. When Freud died in 1940 W. H. Auden wrote: '[Freud] is no more a person now but a whole climate of opinion'.[6] His concepts are probably now more powerful in literary criticism and the arts than in medicine, where they have been subject to some criticism. For example, Karl Popper pointed out that psychoanalysis and Marxism had much in common in that both had an infinitely flexible theoretical basis so that the theory could always be changed to deal with any criticism and thus they should not be considered science. Another view is that Freud's essential role was as a teacher who has taught us to think differently about human behaviour and the way the mind works. Some psychoanalysts abandoned much of Freud's theories in order to develop short-term effective treatments, such as cognitive behavioural therapies. The place of psychoanalysis in medicine was much discussed in the Association – there were many papers on this subject presented at the annual meeting.[7] After the Second World War the majority of psychotherapists in the RMPA were psychoanalysts, which made it difficult for other behavioural methods of psychotherapy to develop in the new College.

---

5   Online archive 25b. Child psychiatry.
6   Auden, W. H. (1940) In Memory of Sigmund Freud. In *Collected Poems* (1976), p. 216. Random House.
7   Notes and News (1921) *JMS*, **67**, 104–123.

The tension between psychodynamic and behavioural and cognitive psychotherapists (BCP) has been present since the development of behaviour therapy in the 1960s. One problem was that BCP had never subscribed to the philosophy that the main purpose of therapy was to elucidate the meaning of symptoms and problems, and to bring unconscious conflicts into consciousness. Another major difference was the emphasis of psychodynamic therapists on personal therapy as part of training – which some BCP therapists considered as potentially detracting from their intellectual independence. Psychotherapists agree on the need for ethical guidelines for practice and the necessity for proper training and supervision. Behavioural and cognitive psychotherapists additionally insist on the need for rigorous evaluation of results, an issue on which some psychodynamic practitioners were ambivalent in the past. The differences between psychoanalysts and behaviourists caused problems, which are discussed in greater detail in the online archives.[8]

Old age psychiatry

Old age psychiatry is one of the younger specialties within psychiatry, and is concerned with the increasing number of older patients suffering from mental disorders with a steadily ageing population. Elderly patients with chronic disorders used to be admitted to asylums (later mental hospitals) and could remain there for life. Generally their conditions were presumed to be irreversible and little treatment as such was available until after the Second World War. Psychiatric care was provided by general psychiatrists rather than specialists up until the 1960s. A College Group for the Psychiatry of Old Age first met in 1973, with Dr Felix Post in the chair.[9]

Changes came about for two reasons. Some general psychiatrists and neuropathologists began to study more closely elderly patients with mental illnesses. Diagnoses and prognoses were clarified. At the same time, with a reduction in the number of hospital beds (particularly in mental hospitals), general psychiatrists found themselves under increasing pressure and were pleased to have colleagues who would take over the responsibility for the elderly. There had been tension between general physicians and psychiatrists about the responsibility for the very elderly who were both physically and mentally handicapped, sometimes following a series of strokes. Initially old age psychiatrists were given responsibility for large numbers of hospital beds, but increasingly their work entailed much more involvement in the community. They were an early group to introduce outreach from the hospital, forming community psychiatric teams with nurses, psychologists, social workers and doctors working very closely with general practitioners.

8   Online archive 25*b*. Psychotherapy.
9   News and Notes (1973), May, 5.

The past 50 years have seen a profound change in the manner in which the elderly with mental disorders are assessed, managed and treated. They are now seen at home or in out-patient clinics much earlier in their illnesses when they can be carefully assessed. Advances in investigation techniques, including neuroimaging, together with raised awareness and expectations within the general population, mean that a combination of community and clinic-based work (sometimes organised as a 'memory clinic') has become standard. Patients and their carers (frequently elderly spouses) are helped by the usual treatments, as well as day care, respite care and financial support. The number of beds in large mental hospitals has dwindled and they have now all but disappeared, while smaller and more appropriate nursing homes, usually private, have greatly increased in number. However, multiple dispersed units present greater problems of surveillance and of regulation of standards. It has become clear that there are some mental disorders in old age, for example the depressions and mental states secondary to treatable physical disorders, which can respond well to specific treatments. There are now drugs that, it is claimed, delay the progression of dementia and these may be succeeded by more effective ones. Even so, much of the work of old age psychiatrists will continue to be providing support to patients and carers.

Substance misuse

In the 1800s psychiatrists thought excessive drinking was one of the causes of mental illness. They also were aware that people could become addicted to alcohol and to other drugs such as opium. This was considered to be due to depravity or weakness of will rather than to an illness. Those whose drinking had badly damaged their brain were cared for in asylums. During and after the First World War the amount of alcohol consumed was very considerably reduced following an increase in price and other controls in the UK introduced by Lloyd George. After the Second World War there was a steady reduction in the real price of alcohol, with increasing consumption and the many harms associated with this. There was also a steady increase in other drugs taken for social and recreational reasons. It became known that tobacco (nicotine), particularly when smoked as cigarettes, was one of the most powerfully addictive of all drugs. The medical profession accepted the idea that addiction (dependence) was an illness and the College established a Dependence/Addiction Group in 1978, at the instigation of the author. This became the Faculty of Substance Misuse in 1997, changing its name to the Addictions Faculty in 2006.[10]

By 2007 there were signs of specialty inflation with the following faculties: Academic, Addictions, Child and Adolescent Psychiatry, Forensic Psychiatry, Liaison Psychiatry, Psychiatry of Learning Disability, Psychiatry of Old Age,

---

10   Online archive 25*b*. Substance misuse.

Psychotherapy, Rehabilitation, Social Psychiatry and Substance Misuse. Perinatal Psychiatry remained as a lone section but many special interest groups were formed, each with their own programme of activities: Adolescent Forensic Psychiatry, Eating Disorders, Gay and Lesbian, Management in Psychiatry, Mental Health Informatics, Neuropsychiatry, Philosophy, Private and Independent Practice, Psychopharmacology, Spirituality, Transcultural Psychiatry and Women in Psychiatry. The History of Psychiatry Special Interest Group became extinct.

CHAPTER 10

Association and College research and the College Research Unit

One of the purposes for which the Association and later the College had been constituted was to 'promote study and research work in psychiatry and all sciences connected with the understanding and treatment of mental disorder in all its forms and aspects and related subjects and publish the results of all such study and research.'[1] Research had always been on the agenda of the Association and the College. Over the years it was recorded on many occasions that the organisation ought to be advocating and carrying out new research and it was promoted by various individuals and institutions (Sir James Crichton-Browne, Leeds University, the Maudsley Hospital and London University). In the late 1980s a small research unit in the College was started. This has proved to be successful in obtaining grants to carry out many multidisciplinary studies into mental illness and in its first 20 years it has published nearly 300 papers. The College is finally carrying out its research remit.

When in 1841 the Association of Medical Officers was founded psychiatrists were aware of the need for research into the mental illnesses. Samuel Hitch, the founder, thought that the members should cooperate in collecting statistical information relating to insanity. At their first meeting they recommended that 'to ensure a correct comparison of the results of treatment, uniform registers [should] be kept and that tabular statements upon a like uniform plan be circulated with the annual report of each hospital'.[2] John Conolly (three times chairman of the Association) spoke strongly of the wealth of case material in hospitals and the need to learn from these through appropriate study and research. Henry Maudsley, one of the main figures of 19th century psychiatry, was always concerned about the paucity of research in the subject and left a substantial sum of money to what later became the Maudsley Hospital and the Institute of Psychiatry. Almost from its inception, the Association and later the MPA and the RMPA all regularly reiterated the view that they should promote and encourage research, yet in practice they could do little. The early research work carried out by Sir James Crichton-Browne and his colleagues in the 'Wakefield triangle' group of hospitals and Leeds University was briefly mentioned in Chapter 4. Similarly, Maudsley, Mott, Mapother and Lewis at

---

1   Supplemental Charter and Bye-laws, Royal College of Psychiatrists 1971, p. 2.
2   Minute Book 1, College archives, 1841.

a later date promoted research at the Maudsley Hospital and the Institute of Psychiatry.

When the College was founded in 1972 further efforts were made which finally resulted in the formation of the College Research Unit in 1987. There also existed a Research Committee who supported the idea of undertaking research projects by the College as this encouraged critical attitudes of mind. They were aware that many junior psychiatrists undertook no research and expressed little interest in it. This appeared to be attributable to preoccupation with other aspects of training and examination, and lack of positive encouragement on the part of some of their seniors. The Committee believed it was important that the College as a whole should be seen to value research and communicate this by example to those entering psychiatry. Suggestions about research had originated from individual members, and from officers and committees of the College, and the Research Committee had undertaken some projects arising from these. Most had been of limited sise and were carried out by individual members with the support of the Committee and the help of the College secretariat.

One of the research projects that had arisen from questions and comments from the Medical Research Council and the Department of Health and Social Services (DHSS) was a survey into the delivery of ECT in 1978, for which a £78 000 grant had been obtained from the DHSS. Dr John Pippard in 1980 studied a cross-section of psychiatric units in two regions. He found standards were abysmally low. Junior psychiatrists who gave the treatments had often not been trained to do this, nor were they supervised. The apparatus used was often obsolete. There was lack of anaesthetic supervision and often there was no adequate resuscitation equipment. This study showed clearly that much was wrong. The College then set up a special working group to lay down minimum standards, give advice, devise guidelines and make provision for further reviews to ensure that standards had been raised. The first review showed that little had changed and that guidelines alone were not enough. More training was essential and equipment needed to be replaced. Stringent review and follow-up of the actions taken led over time to ECT being given only by properly trained and supervised staff. Anaesthesia was provided by qualified doctors in units with proper equipment and standards became strictly controlled. This study turned into a successful continuing audit procedure. Even in its earlier stages the Research Committee believed that it had enhanced the College's prestige.

The Committee wished to see the College more involved in research activities and considered that this could best be done if a research office or unit were established. Their working party drew up a plan recommending that a unit should be sited within the College and closely associated with it. This way, members, officers and secretarial staff would have easy access to it. It was also proposed that the support staff should consist of a non-medical research officer with some knowledge of statistical and computing techniques but not with these exclusively; they would work full time but on a short-term contract. The unit would require clerical and secretarial staff, possibly one person, full-time or part-time and offering about 30 hours per week throughout the year.

John Gunn, who was chairman of the Research Committee from 1977 to 1980, and other members of the Committee, had been strongly in favour of developing such a unit. Their proposal never came to anything at the time as there was significant opposition to it from academic psychiatrists and particularly from senior academics on the staff of the Institute of Psychiatry and Maudsley Hospital. This attitude was not surprising as most of those who opposed the unit had trained at the Institute when Aubrey Lewis was its director. They held the view that all psychiatric research should be based in a university department rather than elsewhere. The president at the time (Professor Kenneth Rawnsley), who had himself trained at the Maudsley and the Institute, was swayed by these arguments. He did not officially disapprove of the idea of a College Research Unit but his support was only lukewarm. Council decided there would be insufficient space in the College for it, despite Sheila Mann (secretary of the Research Committee) believing she had found enough in the unoccupied basement. (She was told that this was earmarked for other uses.) The Research Committee, however, formally proposed forming a research unit to Council, who approved it in principle (it being noted, however, that it was unlikely, at least in the near future, that accommodation would be available at the College headquarters, nor was there money to finance it). The proposal was discussed by the Executive and Finance Committee and quietly shelved. Council had formally agreed to have a research unit but the Executive thought that it should be formed gradually and over a long time. In other words, the proposal would be allowed to wither on the vine. John Gunn resigned as Chairman of the Research Committee ostensibly (according to their minutes) as he had to chair the Academic Board at the Institute.

It was left to the next president (the author) to resolve the problem. He had been off Council after completing five years as dean two years earlier and took the view that there was much research that the College could and ought to do and that all that was necessary was to find sufficient money and space to start the unit. He expected this would rapidly lead to grants for specific research and be self-supporting and also thought it would be possible to make the necessary space within the College. There was a small building in the College garden which had been used by a resident caretaker and his wife, but a non-resident caretaker was all that was necessary. There was already need for more accommodation within the College, which could be provided by putting a further storey on top of the main building and enlarging the garden building. A mansard roof could be added, giving twelve extra spaces and a further storey would considerably enlarge the harden house. This would provide sufficient space that could be used by both the Examinations Department and a small research unit. The president therefore wrote to all College members suggesting they covenant money to develop a Research Unit. Depending on whether they were inceptors, junior members (below consultant), senior members or fellows they were asked to covenant money for a four-year period. He assumed that 10% would respond and this proved to be the case. This appeal brought in enough money to expand both buildings and start the College Research Unit with a director, an assistant and secretarial support. The Unit soon funded itself with grants from projects and became self-sufficient. The first director was Professor John Wing, succeeded by Dr Paul Lelliott. The Unit proved so successful and increased in sise so rapidly that it needed to move to larger rented premises in Grosvenor Crescent in 1995. In 1999 it moved to 83 Victoria Street and in 2005 it had to move yet again to the fourth floor of a modern office block in Aldgate. In 1993 the Unit reported on its first five years of activity:

'The College Research Unit (CRU) had been set up with the aid of funds contributed by College members ... No conditions were laid down as to how the Unit should be run. It was accepted that the director should be responsible for scientific standards and publications and generally for the research strategy, taking into account College needs. Officers also accepted that its agenda and staff must be multidisciplinary. The broad aims set out in the initial application for audit funds were to provide agreed clinical guidelines, recommendations on the structure of district services relative to population need, methods of data collection in clinical practice from which useful district and national information could be drawn, and a central information base and advisory centre. The last of these aims was conceptualised as an office that would serve to act as a means of two-way communication between the CRU, on the one hand, and College officers, department heads and the membership more generally, on the other .The CRU contribution would be concentrated particularly on research and technical issues associated with clinical audit and information systems. By a happy chance, John Pippard was available to repeat the survey of ECT administration that he had undertaken several years earlier and which had led to the promulgation of College guidelines. In this case, "completing the audit cycle" demonstrated that guidelines, even if correct, were useless if not acted upon, a lesson that both the College and its Research Unit found salutary. The College has taken a range of actions aimed at remedying the position and the CRU is about to repeat the survey. This is research linked to practical clinical audit.'

When the CRU moved from the College building to 11 Grosvenor Crescent it had become multidisciplinary, with staff from a variety of backgrounds including psychiatry, nursing, psychology, service management and health economics. At that time it had funding for eight research and development and seven secretarial and administrative staff. There were further four staff working on affiliated projects for which the Unit was the grant holder.

The CRU had reviewed the challenges to mental healthcare. These included lack of information, inadequate and unbalanced provision of services, poor communication, and low morale. Further information was needed to help mental health workers decide which type of intervention best suited individual patients and to help planners decide how to reconfigure services to meet the needs of their catchment population. Mental health services had undergone a rapid transformation from being centred on large-scale asylums to focus on care in the community. Three-quarters of all psychiatric hospital beds had closed during the previous 40 years. However, there had not been an equivalent investment in alternative services and there was severe pressure on the existing ones, especially those in inner cities. In particular, psychiatric admission beds and high-staffed hostel places were in short supply. Some disabled people with mental illness were being cared for outside hospital. It was vital to their well-being, and sometimes to their or the others' safety that those delivering care communicated effectively. Enquiries had consistently identified difficulties in communication, particularly between health and social services, as a factor contributing to highly publicised incidents involving people with mental illness. As mental health services adapted to the changes, mental health professionals were working in an increasingly demanding environment. Reviews showed a high incidence of stress and low morale among all groups. Many mental health services had serious difficulty in recruiting staff, including psychiatrists.

The CRU worked to help mental health services meet those challenges. Three strands to its programme of work can be identified:

- clinical audit and quality – developing standards for care and for organisations and the means of implementing these;
- information strategy, systems and technology – improving the quality of information about the process and outcomes of mental healthcare, and the ways in which this information is used and communicated;
- health services research – identifying the necessary components and structure of an effective mental health service.

The CRU recognised that joint working was an important element in the effective delivery of care and, as a reflection of this, its staff have come from a variety of professional backgrounds. In addition, the Unit had established close working links with research and development organisations that represented a range of disciplines. It works with a large number of services and professionals across the UK and, whenever possible and appropriate, involves service users. The CRU believes that for its work to have real value it must be capable of local implementation. To fulfil this aim the CRU offers training to professionals, support to services in evaluating their effectiveness, and produces audit and evaluation tools which can be used locally.

Research methods training

At the time the Research Unit was set up it was considered that it would be desirable to improve research methods training for both senior registrars (later specialist psychiatric registrars) and newly appointed consultants. From the mid-1980s to the mid-1990s Chris Freeman and Peter Tyrer regularly ran research methods workshops under the auspices of the Research Committee, travelling to all parts of the country to do this (including a notable conference in Cork where a trainee from Yorkshire, drunk on red wine, vomited over a nun's carpet, causing the College to receive a bill for several thousand pounds worth of damages). By the mid-1990s most training schemes had incorporated research methods training into their curriculum and the research methods course is now a twice yearly event held in Leeds.

Publications

The CRU has published nearly 300 papers in its years of existence. A full list is available from the College and the CRU website.

The College Research Unit has been a success which can now carry out Samuel Hitch's hopes by promoting research and cooperate in collecting statistical information relating to insanity, among their other responsibilities. Through the CRU the College is now promoting study and research work in psychiatry.[3]

---

3   Online archive 25c. The College Research Unit today.

CHAPTER 11

Education and training of nurses

Asylum superintendents were aware from early days of the important role of 'attendants' or nurses, but it was not until the 1870s that the MPA showed interest in this matter. From then on, it developed training, examinations and a register which continued for many years until those functions were taken over by national nursing bodies. This chapter borrows very heavily from an article by Dr Alexander Walk on the history of mental nursing.[1]

The early role of nurses

The involvement of the MPA in the education of nurse attendants formally started in 1883, although as early as 1817 in his work *Moral Management* J. Haslam had described the depressed state of the occupation of 'keeper'.[2] He emphasised the keeper's need for careful and sympathetic direction by the physician in charge of the case and pointed out the severe handicaps under which the staff worked, especially through their insufficient numbers. In the Bethlem Hospital, before 1815, there were only five attendants for 120 male patients, and two for 66 female patients. Haslam urged 'some plan to improve the condition of the keeper' and made two suggestions – 'the establishment of a fund, and a provision for the later period of their lives, to which during their employment they should contribute', and the formation of 'a register of persons calculated to officiate as keepers – an essential service to the public and the medical profession'. In 1796 the newly opened Retreat appointed a matron or 'female superintendent', Katherine Allen, and she and her husband, the first 'superintendent' or chief male nurse, George Jepson, may be regarded as one of the first nurses credited with promoting moral treatment. In the *Sketch of the Retreat* (1828) George Jepson is given the credit for the introduction of some of the methods of moral treatment.[3]

A different example of the work of a married couple was provided shortly afterwards at Wakefield Asylum (now Stanley Royd Hospital), in the same

---

1   Walk, A. (1961) The history of mental nursing. *JMS*, **107**, 1–17.

2   Haslam, J. (1817) *Considerations on the Moral Management of Insane Persons.* pp. 32–39. Hunter.

3   *A Sketch of the Origin, Progress and Present State of the Retreat* (1828). (Anonymous, sometimes attributed to Samuel Tuke).

county. Wakefield, which opened in 1818, was a conscious attempt to apply Retreat principles to a county asylum of 150–200 beds. The magistrates had appointed as superintendent Dr (later Sir) William Ellis, and continued the practice of naming the physician superintendent's wife as the matron. Ellis's *Treatise on Insanity*, published in 1838, gave numerous examples of his wife's skill and readiness of wit in handling difficult patients. It was her idea to introduce the making of fancy articles, suited to the patients' tastes, and sold to the public at a permanent 'bazaar' within the hospital.

There are no grounds for the assumption that the term 'nurse' indicated a more therapeutic rôle than the others. The words 'keeper', 'attendant', 'nurse' and sometimes 'superintendent' were used indifferently except that 'nurse' was generally confined to women. This is shown in a passage from John Conolly's *Indications of Insanity* (1830). 'Every patient,' he said 'should have a superintendent or keeper with him during a great part of each day, so long as there remains a hope of cure. Every opportunity should be taken of effecting the restoration of the patient to mental health ... to converse with, to amuse, to instruct the patients, is the great business of each day.'[4] He used the terms 'attendants', 'nurses' and 'staff' interchangeably. To enable the non-restraint system to be followed in its completeness meant regulating every word, look and action of all who come in contact with the insane. Conolly insisted on personally selecting candidates and had no difficulty in recruiting from 'the class of persons qualified to be upper servants', given a fair remuneration and a prospect of comfort. He did not expect to be allowed more than one attendant to about 15 patients, though his wish was for one to five, as in private asylums. Their duties, he said, began early, were incessant during the day, and ended late. These duties he described in minute detail, without at any time allowing the reader to forget the spirit in which they were meant to be carried out. Conolly noted that Dr Gaskell of Lancaster employed night attendants with few or no day duties and by this means had got the better of the uncleanly habits of almost every patient.

Conolly's matron at Hanwell, Miss Powell, was a loyal supporter of his reforms; her successor held a similar post with W. A. F. Browne at Montrose. But in general both Conolly and subsequent medical authors in the Association's Journal and elsewhere expressed critical opinions about the matrons, who had been entrusted with, or assumed powers for which they were in no way fitted by training or experience, and were said to use those powers to hamper progress. Over the next forty years the general opinion was that a 'chief nurse' promoted from the ranks was preferable to an amateur 'lady matron'. Clarification of the duties of a matron came much later when as a professional hospital-trained nurse she was seen to be an essential leader in the movement for what was called the 'hospitalisation of the asylums'.

Later, between 1845 and 1860, it became difficult to recruit staff with the required mental and moral qualities as the expansion of the asylum

---

4   Conolly, J. (1830) *The Indications of Insanity.* (reprinted 1964). p. 487. Dawsons.

service was rapid, and the increased demand too great. When in 1854 the Commissioners in Lunacy called for reports from all the hospitals under their jurisdiction, only the smaller ones were able to describe a satisfactory state of affairs. They continued to stress the importance of improving the nurses' and attendants' conditions of work, their remuneration and status. From 1857 onwards they recorded and commended the system of separate night nursing, although it is clear this existed in only a rudimentary form.

Arlidge's book *On the State of Lunacy* (1859) included a thorough discussion of the attendant problem. He pointed out that among many other handicaps, the attendants 'have no preliminary instruction or training, but have to learn their duties in the exercise of them … Many are their failures, yet on the whole, considering their antecedents and the nature of the duties imposed on them, their success is remarkable.'[5] Arlidge made the constructive suggestion that the system then adopted in the large London hospitals should be extended to the asylums, whereby the office of 'sister' to nurse the patients should be separated from that of 'under-nurse' to whom the cleanliness of the ward was committed.

Conolly must have attempted to train his staff by personal precept and practice. Hack Tuke's *Dictionary of Psychological Medicine*[6] mentions Conolly's work 'Teachings for Attendant', but this has not been traced. W. H. O. Sankey, Conolly's successor at Hanwell, quoted from a booklet of instructions which he had prepared to supplement the statutory *Manual of Duties*. Conolly's high ideal of 'regulating every word, look and action of all who come in contact with the insane' is fully supported there.

Lectures

The beginnings of mental nurse training preceded the giving of a formal course of lectures. The first known set of lectures to mental nurses were those given by Sir Alexander Morison at the Surrey Asylum (later Springfield Hospital), in 1843–1844. Morison, who had given the first lectures on insanity to students in Edinburgh twenty years earlier, was visiting physician to Springfield. He pointed out to the attendants the means by which they could acquire the patients' regard and confidence and could induce them to occupy themselves in useful employments and rational amusements. Morison was one of the founders of the Society for Improving the Condition of the Insane, and several of his hospital staff obtained 'premiums' offered by the Society as rewards for 'meritorious conduct.' There is no evidence that these lectures were ever established as a permanent feature.

Another ephemeral venture was that of W. A. F. Browne at the Crichton Royal Hospital in 1854. In 1837, his book *What Asylums Were, Are and Ought To Be* called for some system of instruction for attendants and praised the

5   Arlidge, J. T. (1859) *On the State of Lunacy and the Legal Provision for the Insane*. John Churchill.
6   Tuke, D. H. (ed.) (1892) *A Dictionary of Psychological Medicine*. J. & A. Churchill.

apprenticeship scheme in force in some French asylums.[7] In 1854 Browne gave a course of thirty lectures, primarily to the officers and attendants, but also to some of the patients who belonged to the medical profession. The lectures viewed mental illness from various angles, for example as the relation of the insane to the community, to their friends and custodians. Treatment, so far as it depended upon external impressions and the influence of sound mind, was discussed. Browne attempted to impart instruction by examples drawn from actual inmates.

The interest of the Association in the training of nurses can be traced from the reports of its meetings in the *Journal of Mental Science*, which by the 1870s showed an increasing interest in asylum attendants. In 1870 a letter, signed 'Asylum Chaplain', appeared in the *Journal* advocating a systematic training of attendants.[8] It suggested that the MPA should authorise some qualified persons to write a simple catechism embodying what was required of an efficient attendant. Novices were to be tested, and until they had passed through this ordeal they should be regarded as simply probationers. According to Dr Walk, the author was probably the Rev. Henry Hawkins of Colney Hatch, who later founded the Mental After-Care Association. There was no immediate response to his proposal.

Clouston's paper and the debate that ensued

Dr Thomas Clouston, who was physician-superintendent of the Royal Edinburgh Asylum, addressed the MPA annual meeting in 1876 on getting, training and retaining good asylum attendants.[9] Clouston dwelt at length on the constantly shifting population of inexperienced attendants, on the need for natural aptitude and the unpredictability of success in the work. He outlined his methods of personal and individual training. He advocated the use of a special 'hospital ward' in which all new attendants would be trained. There would be in charge a person of intelligence and experience who would instruct the novices in the routine ward work. One of the medical officers would spend some time each day showing them the peculiarities and habits characteristic of particular mental illnesses, drafting in for this purpose a typical suicidal melancholic, an acutely excited patient, a general paralytic and so on; the novice would be given charge of each of these in succession and be made to walk, work, and eat with him. The doctor and the chief attendant would examine the novice and teach him every day about things to be known and done. The novice should accompany their patients during the visits of the relatives, to try and find out why and how the disease arose. Lectures, once a week in the winter evenings, were to supplement this

---

7   Browne, W. A. F. (1837) *What Asylums Were, Are and Ought To Be*. Adam and Charles Black.

8   An Asylum Chaplain (1870) Attendants in Asylums. *JMS*, **16**, 310–311.

9   Clouston, T. S. (1876) On the question of getting, training and retaining the services of good asylum attendants. *JMS*, **22**, 381–388.

practical teaching. Clouston added a number of suggestions for improving the conditions under which attendants worked to boost their morale. His methods of nurse training were essentially practical and 'patient-centred'. He believed in the separate and distinctive 'hospital ward,' and it was through his influence and that of his English pupil Hayes Newington that the detached hospital unit, either for the sick or for short-term admissions, became a common feature of asylums. His enthusiasm for hospital features went further, and the approximation of the methods of the asylum to those of the general hospital was regarded as an aim in itself. The discussion on Clouston's paper showed that his recommendations were warmly supported, but little was said on training, the main subject of his address. A small committee was formed to report on the advisability of forming an 'association' or 'registry' of attendants in connection with the MPA, but nothing appears to have come of this.

Another six years' silence followed this debate, broken only by grumbles (in asylum and Commissioners' annual reports) about 'frequent changes in the staff', or the difficulty of keeping out 'undesirable attendants'. Then at the MPA quarterly meeting in Edinburgh in 1883 Campbell Clark, of the district asylum, Bothwell, read a paper which led directly to the developments of the next few years – 'The special training of asylum attendants'.[10] Clark had been encouraged to start a course of teaching by the zeal and thirst for information he had found among some of his staff. His first course, in 1882, he felt was only a partial success, as he thought that many of the lectures had been aimed too high. His second course was simpler and more practical, and he felt that he had hit the right nail on the head. Concurrently he gave ward teaching, and at the end of the course prizes were offered for essays on a subject such as 'hallucinations'. Apart from that, the attendants held informal club meetings, at which the lectures and their application to particular patients were discussed, and thus a kind of 'mental improvement society' was established.

The MPA 1883 meeting resolved that, 'a committee of the medical officers of the asylums of Scotland be appointed for the purpose of considering the questions of (1) the special training and instruction of asylum attendants and the best modes of doing so and (2) the preparation of a manual of instructions for nursing and attendance on the insane'.[11] A committee was then nominated consisting of all present, numbering about a dozen. Clark revealed considerable respect for attendants and expressed the view that 'too great a barrier existed between officers and attendants and that the mental and moral qualities of attendants were not utilised as fully as they might have been and that attendants required to be individualised as well as patients'.[12] He further described the contemporary status of attendants and emphasised the importance of training and recruitment. Clark encouraged

10   Clark, A. C. (1884) The special training of asylum attendants. *JMS*, **29**, 459–466.
11   Notes and News (1884) *JMS*, **30**, 162.
12   Clark, A. C. (1884) The special training of asylum attendants. *JMS*, **29**, 459–466.

the MPA to endorse his pioneering steps and to foster attendant training generally. He conveyed a sense of urgency for change since 'knowledge of insanity and its appropriate treatment is growing apace'.[13] He drew attention to changing asylum practice, particularly the trend towards 'individualising' patients, but he made clear that 'the attendants are not sufficiently trained and elevated to fit into the new order of things ... If our asylums are to be more like hospitals, our attendants, like hospital nurses, must be specially trained.'[14]

The handbook

The outcome of the meeting was a Handbook and Training of Attendants Committee. This worked quickly and proofs of the *Handbook for the Instruction of Attendants on the Insane* were shown to the MPA quarterly meetings in 1884. It was accepted for print and it was decided that 1000 copies would be distributed. The handbook was first published in 1885 as a slim volume, bound in red hardboard, and consisted of 64 pages of text together with an appendix listing all the public and private lunatic asylums in the UK and their superintendents. It was divided into five chapters:

I   The body, its general functions and disorders
II   The nursing of the sick
III Mind and its disorders
IV   The care of the insane
V   The general duties of attendants

In 1885, the Journal published a review of the book: 'We are not quite sure ourselves whether it is necessary or wise to attempt to convey instructions in physiology etc., to ordinary attendants. Will they be the better equipped for their duties for being told that the brain consists of grey and white matter and cement substance? We hardly see what is to be gained by superficial knowledge of this kind.'[15] Considering the book's brevity and the ambitious scope of its contents, it is not surprising that the information it contained was of necessity condensed and elementary. The handbook served as an important milestone in the history of the education of 'attendants on the insane', who must previously have been regarded as little more than pairs of hands. The labours of a Glasgow subcommittee of the Scottish Division were fully justified, and were reflected in the success which the handbook and its successors enjoyed in the century following the original publication. The many editions attempted to keep pace with developments in the field and contained a condensed history of British psychiatry.[16]

The handbook was always published in conjunction with the MPA, and later the RMPA, though over the years it changed in title and format. The

---

13   ibid.
14   ibid.
15   Instruction of Attendants (1885) *JMS*, **31**, 149.
16   Online archive 25*a*. Divisions.

7th edition, published in 1923, was renamed the *Handbook for Mental Nurses*, but it was known more familiarly by generations of psychiatric nurses as 'the red handbook'.

In April 1964, the 9th edition appeared under the editorship of Brian Ackner, who enlisted psychiatrists, a senior psychiatric social worker and a superintendent of nursing. There were 335 pages of text, a suggested reading list, and a glossary of terms. This edition was reprinted six times, the last of which was in June 1978. In 1979, the Education Committee of the College concluded that the book was out of date and decided not to commission a further edition. They thought future textbooks should be written by nurses themselves.[17]

Nursing exams

Five years elapsed between the publication of the first handbook and the first examinations. The MPA meeting reports for the late 1880s contain some references to lectures and teaching in nursing in mental healthcare and in 1889 Dr Campbell Clark spoke of his own examinations for attendants. Once more the MPA appointed a committee, this time to inquire into the possibility of organising systematic training of nurses and attendants in asylums, which soon recommended that attendants should have two years of training followed by the MPA examinations. The MPA would also issue certificates and keep a register. The Education Committee's scheme for a nursing proficiency certificate was accepted at the 1890 annual meeting and the first examinations (for the Certificare of Proficiency in Nursing) were held the following year. To consider the business of the examinations and keep the register of those who had passed, a new office of registrar was created in 1892. Dr Beveridge Spence of Lichfield was appointed to this post.

The examinations became established rapidly. In 1899 Dr Spence was elected president of the MPA and reviewed what had been achieved up to that point in his presidential address.[18] By 1898 over 100 asylums were participating and between 500 and 600 certificates were granted every year. In the light of experience, modifications had been introduced; written answers were now marked independently from oral examinations, and the external examiner took a larger part in the oral examinations. Certain certificated nurses from general hospitals were allowed to qualify in one year.

The MPA took its nursing examinations seriously and, despite not having a permanent headquarters or paid staff, retained records of their administration, which was the responsibility of the standing Education

---

17   Rollin, H. R. (1986) The Red Handbook: An historic centenary. *Bulletin of the Royal College of Psychiatrists*, **10**, 279.

18   Presidential Address (1899) *JMS*, **45**, 635–657.

Committee. This committee was first appointed in 1893 when the MPA was planning its own qualification for doctors, but the attendants' examinations quickly became a large part of its work. It met three or four times a year, and its reports and the reports of the MPA Council regularly recorded the appointment of other committees to deal with specific training matters.

The extension of training from 2 to 3 years was first recommended in 1897 and began in 1906 with a preliminary examination in 1908. There was considerable discussion in the 1920s about the length of training and the precise nature of nursing qualifications. The position of nurses with elements of general training entering mental nurse training and the relative position of asylum and hospital trained nurses became a point of issue with the General Nursing Council (GNC).

Before the end of the 19th century, the MPA considered extending its examinations abroad, first to South Africa in 1892 and then to other British colonies and overseas. It was agreed in 1903 that the MPA certificate would not be promoted in areas where training and examinations had already been established. Candidates from South Africa were soon admitted and South African examinations began in 1921. The MPA began to consider the recognition of examinations then being held in southern Australia and this matter became part of wider discussion on setting up colonial branches – a regular, if infrequent, suggestion that never became a reality. Help with examinations for a mental hospital in Canada was authorised in 1926 and in 1920 Danish trained nurses were recognised. This was possibly the only time European qualifications were recognised by the MPA, although parts of the handbook had been translated into French when the French were developing their own training systems.

The hospitalisation movement

General hospital-trained nurses were brought in as matrons of asylums. In order to give them some experience of the care of mental patients, they were usually first appointed as assistant matrons with a view to promotion at an early date. In a number of Scottish asylums the matron was given control of both the male and female wards in the hospital. These measures may have contributed to raising the standard of bedside nursing; yet they could not fail also to lower the status of the mental nurse and to confirm and strengthen the bias away from the principles of moral treatment. The matrons and assistant matrons recruited in small numbers at Edinburgh and elsewhere were women of superior intelligence and education, and it was this rather than the mere possession of a certificate of general training that was the reason for their success.

Another aspect of the 'hospitalisation movement' was the spread of the nursing of male patients by female nurses. Historically, the use of women nurses in this way was in its origins a method of moral treatment; for, like a number of other original and unconventional measures, it was first practised in the 1840s by Samuel Hitch in Gloucester, and the married couple whom he employed were in charge of the refractory, not the infirmary ward. Maudsley in 1868 pointed out that a deluded and hostile patient would yield to a woman's persuasion more readily and with less feeling of humiliation, and in the same year Crichton-Browne at Wakefield successfully introduced a woman nurse as an auxiliary into a ward of seventy epileptic and suicidal patients. After various other experiments, George Robertson, by his writings and practice at Perth, Stirling and Edinburgh, did much to secure a general acceptance of the principle; combining it as he did with the introduction of the general hospital-trained nurse, he was able to show impressive results in the improved habits and behaviour of turbulent patients as well as better nursing in the sick wards. The shortage of male staff during the First World War led to a still wider spread of female nursing, and by the year 1925 there were few hospitals where at least one or two male infirmary wards were not staffed by women. Such policy was later violently attacked by the Asylum Workers' Union as a cunning conspiracy to secure cheap labour. It is evident that this was not the motive that inspired Hitch or Crichton-Browne or George Robertson, or that impelled the Boards of Control to give their support.

At the Retreat, Dr Bedford Pierce set an example of mental nurse training on progressive lines. The hospital's duty was to provide training and in return probationers entered into a four-year contract. The status of the charge nurses, here called ward sisters, was raised, and ward instruction was given by them and by the matron. Pierce stressed the need for the training of the nurse's personal habits and powers, her social gifts and accomplishments, as well as proficiency in certain physical methods of treatment – for such methods existed and were much valued even in 1903. He looked forward to better cooperation between the hospitals for the sick and for the insane, which should be on equal terms. The collected *Addresses to Mental Nurses* delivered annually at the Retreat by distinguished guest speakers over a number of years and edited by Bedford Pierce, in 1921 recorded the principles and ideals which they sought to instil. In the same year Pierce was appointed one of the first psychiatric members of the newly created General Nursing Council for England and Wales and chairman of its Mental Nursing Committee.

A separate examination for the nurses of 'mental defectives' (i.e. people with learning disability, as they were then known) was first suggested in 1896 and again in 1917, and the first such examination was set in 1918. Further examinations for attendants of mental deficiency hospitals and a diploma in training medical officers in mental deficiency institutions were discussed in the 1920s and 1930s but were not developed. Much of the administration was covered by the existing regulations and was carried out by the Mental Deficiency Committee, the forerunner of the College's present Faculty for Learning Disability. In 1939, half the committees reporting to Council were concerned with training and examinations, a reflection of the amount of work (all voluntary) that was involved.

The nursing badge

At first, the names of successful candidates were printed in the *Journal of Mental Science*. They were issued with a certificate and entitled to a badge or medal (the terms seem to have been used interchangeably). After 1918, certificates were no longer issued to successful candidates in the preliminary examinations; instead, to avoid them using the certificate to claim full qualifications, their names were entered on a register. Final certificates continued to be issued. The first Nursing Badge Committee was appointed in 1893 and the design they agreed on showed Psyche, representing the soul or spirit. In 1903 the Education Committee gave figures for the issue of badges and medals and agreed they would be engraved with the recipient's name instead of their number. Six years later it was agreed that the words 'with distinction' would be added where appropriate. In 1926 the design was changed when the MPA received its Royal Charter and Psyche was replaced by the newly acquired coat of arms. At the same time, the addition of an optional ribbon was approved – blue to correspond with the colour in the president's badge of office. In 1928 an additional badge to be worn on outdoor uniform was suggested. The same year, after much discussion, an honorary nursing medal and certificate was presented to Princess Mary, who had shown a keen interest in nurses' training and welfare. The RMPA tried hard to retain its own examinations despite a 'revolutionary' resolution submitted by the Scottish Division in 1937, suggesting that they should be abandoned in favour of the GNC's. However, in 1945 the Athlone Committee recommended they should end and the Council reported that relations with the GNC were improving; an agreement was reached in 1946. The RMPA received letters of complaint and regret and the related loss of revenue from fees and the handbook was criticised, but the last nursing examinations were held in 1951.

In 1952, the registrar, Dr Iveson Russell of York, informed the Council that a total of 50 021 Mental Nursing and 5256 Mental Deficiency Nursing Certificates had been issued and there had been no year since 1891 when the examinations had not been held. He continued,

'the Association could look back on this work with some pride. The services involved more than the organisation of examinations at a time when no other branch of nursing had any other national standard or qualification. It standardised the syllabus of training in all the mental hospitals and mental deficiency hospitals of the country, and was almost entirely responsible for the training of mental nurses before the passing of the Nurses' Registration Act in 1919.'[19]

The RMPA also briefly ran an occupational therapy examination. Planning began in the 1930s and there were five successful candidates in 1939. Although the RMPA put its view to the post-war Rushcliffe Committee that

---

19   Council minutes (1952) College archives.

occupational therapy was a nursing duty and tried to revive this examination it was abolished in 1947.

State registration of nurses

The movement for state registration of nurses was originated by Mrs Bedford Fenwick in 1889, and its first instrument was the Royal British Nurses' Association, but for many years the issue was bedevilled by dissensions and splits, and the whole principle of registration was violently opposed, chiefly by certain of the London teaching hospitals. The Royal British Nurses Association was for long time governed by a mixed council of doctors and nurses, and this included several MPA members, notably Sir James Crichton-Browne, Dr Outterson Wood and Professor Ernest White. In 1897 Wood brought the position to the notice of the MPA. He had proposed that nurses holding the MPA's certificate should be recognised as eligible to become members of the Royal British Nurses Association (RBNA) on certain conditions and as a distinct class. In spite of much opposition and a display of prejudice against the asylum trained nurse in one of the nursing journals, the proposal was accepted by the RBNA Council and an alliance was suggested between the two bodies, the MPA conducting the examinations and the RBNA registering the successful candidates on its voluntary register after enquiring into their character and antecedents. Nothing seems to have come of these negotiations. In 1904 rival bills for the state registration of nurses came before Parliament and were both rejected. Instead, a Select Committee was appointed to consider the question and make recommendations. One of the bills provided for a single psychiatric representative on a General Nursing Council of 21, who might be either a doctor or a nurse, and who would be appointed by the Asylum Workers Association. Outterson Wood devoted a large part of his presidential address in 1905 to the subject, and to strengthen the mental nurses' case the training period was lengthened to three years; it was also at about this time that the term 'male nurse' came into general use in place of 'attendant'. At the Select Committee, Ernest White gave evidence of the nature and scope of the MPA examinations, and the Committee (which included among its members Sir John Batty Tuke, the former medical superintendent of the Fife and Kinross asylum and pioneer of the open-door system) recommended that state registration should be instituted and that the MPA examinations should be recognised as qualifying for registration.

In 1895 some MPA members had founded a voluntary organisation named the Asylum Workers Association which was intended to cater for the needs of nurses and attendants. It met for a time with a good deal of success, and in 1905 numbered between 3000 and 4000 members. But its constitution and government were entirely paternal; the secretary was for long Dr Shuttleworth, of the Royal Albert Institution, and the annual meetings, regularly reported in the MPA Journal, consisted largely of uplifting speeches by distinguished honorary vice-presidents; no mental nurse seems ever to have spoken and it is doubtful if any attended. Nevertheless the Asylum Workers Association was certainly moved by a genuine desire to 'improve the professional status of the mental nurse'. It took part in urging the mental nurse's claims to a place in any state registration scheme, and more importantly it actively promoted the plan for a national system of pensions for nursing and other staff, which was embodied in the Asylums Officers' Superannuation Act 1909. It was the passage of this Act that brought to a head the grievances felt by many of the staff, and led in 1910 to the formation of the National Asylum Workers' Union. As the original manifesto of the Union explained, the Act had many imperfections. In particular, exception was taken to the compulsory deductions from wages already too small; but there were deeper grievances. The manifesto contained some notable passages – 'Our minds are not improved, because the conditions of our labour are such that they shut us off from the wider range of Humanity and of books ... apart from any true education we cannot attain to any real moral greatness.' The attitude of most MPA members to this was at first adverse because of an apparent absence on the Union's part of any kind of professional outlook. During its first years the pages of the Union's magazine contained no references to the training or professional status of the mental nurse, although these were the years when attention in the nursing world was constantly focused on these matters. It was not till 1919, when the Nurses' Registration Bill was passed, that the Union first included in its programme a demand for better training facilities in all asylums, and in the same year it successfully claimed the right to be consulted by the Minister of Health and to put forward candidates for seats on the general nursing councils.

In 1916 on the formation of the College of Nursing, the MPA urged upon that body the need for including on its Council people familiar with asylum training, but the College declined. However, when the Nurses' Registration Act was passed in 1919, provision was made for the inclusion of 'nurses trained in the nursing and care of persons suffering from mental diseases' in a Supplementary Part of the Register. For the first English General Nursing Council, the Minister of Health was to make five appointments representative among other things of 'special nursing services and medical practice', and 16 appointments of nurses after consultation with 'associations or organised bodies of nurses'. When the General Nursing Council for England and Wales first met in May 1920, it had among its members one mental hospital physician, Bedford Pierce, appointed by the Minister on the MPA's recommendation, and one mental nurse, Mr Christian of Banstead, appointed on the nomination of the Union. A Standing Committee which included these two members was appointed to consider the position of holders of the MPA certificate, and it was resolved to accept this, during the period of grace, as evidence of training; the recently-established Certificate for Nursing in Mental Deficiency was also accepted. In 1922 it was agreed that holders of the MPA certificate should be eligible for a shortened period of training in general hospitals. For a time it was thought that the GNC for England and Wales might take over the final examination in mental nursing only, leaving the MPA to continue the intermediate examinations, but in 1923 it decided to insist on a common preliminary examination for all nurses. In the same year a joint conference was held between the GNC, the MPA and the Board of Control. It was there stated on behalf of the Council that it had realised that mental nurses would for a considerable time to come prefer not to register and therefore the MPA examination and certificate would be necessary as before. The assistance of the MPA was welcomed and it was invited to nominate examiners and to appoint an advisory committee to the GNC. However, during subsequent years this committee ceased to be consulted, and if the ever-militant Mrs Bedford Fenwick, writing in the *British Journal of Nursing*, is to be believed, the GNC's own Mental Nurses' Committee itself rarely met. So an estrangement between Council and Association began, which lasted for some 20 years. Much of what the MPA did in a fruitless effort to defeat the GNC's policy was misguided, but it maintained the examination in being and eventually led to entry to the register for a large number of nurses who would otherwise have remained unrecognised.

In 1954 a committee was appointed to consider the shortage of mental nurses and the possibility of starting RMPA examinations again, but this came to nothing. For a while, too, the RMPA and GNC needed to work together on disciplinary matters as an RMPA nurse, if struck off the GNC register, could still in theory use the title 'nurse'. To overcome this problem in 1962 it was agreed that the GNC would take over all disciplinary matters and put in place unifying procedures for registration and discipline.

Further reading

Walk, A. (1961) The history of mental nursing. *Journal of Mental Science*, **107**, 1–17.

Parry-Jones, W. (1984) The foundations of psychiatric nurse training. *Bulletin of the Royal College of Psychiatrists*, **8**, 82–83.

CHAPTER 12

Doctors and medical students
Education, training and examination

For many years, the Association did not develop adequate education or training for doctors who worked with the mentally ill. Medical schools in universities were equally slow to provide adequate clinical experience of the mentally ill or knowledge of mental illnesses. Only after the World War II did all medical schools (now departments of universities) start to teach psychiatry, following the recommendations of the Goodenough Committee. Education of psychiatrists became the responsibility of the Royal College of Psychiatrists in the 1970s with the development of methods to monitor and assess all training, teaching and postgraduate education.

Better education and training of doctors in psychological medicine was always the Association's aspiration, but this was not provided till much later than education for keepers and nurses. Asylum doctors (mostly after 1828) were not required to have had any specialist training or any knowledge beyond what every licensed doctor might know in any case. They were quite likely to describe themselves as 'surgeon' in the *Medical Directory*, short for surgeon-apothecary, which indicated general basic qualifications such as Licentiate of the Society of Apothecaries (LSA), and membership of the Royal College of Surgeons (MRCS). There was no formal systematic training either in the diagnosis and treatment of mental disorder, or in hospital administration. The asylum doctor learned on the job, from his senior, if any, and from books and journals. Being employed as a generalist, he was not there to find new cures, or do research, or teach, but to organise physical care. He found himself treating physical ills and teaching attendants how to nurse, helping the epileptic to breathe, the paralytic to eat without inhaling food or vomit, and the bedridden to turn. In the interests of preventive medicine doctors saw to the hospital diet, the fresh air and exercise, the avoidance of cold draughts, and the overcrowding that patients increasingly experienced. Asylum doctors, apart from those working in private hospitals, had no say in who was to be admitted to their asylum: in general, they did no clinical work outside its bounds, and their practical experience of mental illness was limited to what they saw in the asylums they worked in. Some patients recovered, but apart from maintaining physical health and preventing suicide, it was not clear that their treatments had much to do with it. From years of experience, asylum doctors learned administration and something of the ways of the mentally ill. They became specialists as 'alienists'.

There were marked differences in the teaching of psychological medicine in various countries. In England and Ireland the development of the asylum system was separated from general medicine. In Germany in the 19th century, medicine was a university subject that the state was interested in promoting. Able doctors aspired to be university professors, in the specialties as well as in general medicine and surgery, and they usually had hospital wards and consulting rooms where they could demonstrate cases to students and conduct research. Most of the 19th century advances in medicine took place in Germany and Austria, and practice in those countries was generally of a high standard. The teaching and education of psychiatrists was the universities' responsibility. It was a century later that this was adopted in the UK, though there had been occasional attempts to provide some psychiatric education for doctors and medical students.

The Association's concern that doctors should have a better knowledge of mental disorders dates back to its earliest years. It was most notably voiced by Conolly in his presidential address in 1858 and again in 1860. He wished a course of clinical instruction to be compulsory for all asylum medical officers, and urged the newly formed General Medical Council to include insanity in the medical curriculum. The 1862 debate on the future of Bethlem was largely concerned with the possibility of developing the teaching of psychiatry at a rebuilt hospital.

Asylum education

In 1753 the governors of St Luke's Hospital authorised the physician to that hospital to take pupils, though this permission was rescinded 50 years later. By the time the resumption of teaching was authorised in 1843, other places had instituted similar courses. In 1823 Alexander Morison began to give lectures on psychiatry in Edinburgh, which continued in various guises for 20 years. At Hanwell, clinical teaching was commenced by John Conolly in 1842. His account of it years later indicated how much it was linked in his mind with the reforms for which he is now chiefly known:

'It appears to me that then only (i.e. after the abolition of mechanical restraint) could the proper study of insanity begin; the removal of restraints and of all violent and irritating methods of control thus first permitting the students to contemplate disorders of the mind in their simplicity, and no longer modified by exasperating treatment. Patients could then be presented to their observation as subjects of study and reflection ... and regarded as persons to be cured of illness, or relieved from distress, and not as beings to be tortured by confinement of the limbs or mortified, by punishments.'[1]

---

1   Conolly, J. R. (1856) *The Treatment of the Insane without Mechanical Restraints.* (1973) pp. 282–283. Dawson's.

The year after Conolly started his lectures, Bethlem admitted some pupils and from 1848 onwards there were regular courses there lasting for four months and held twice a year.

Students were also admitted to the West Riding Wakefield Asylum, where James Browne was superintendent from 1866 to 1876. He founded and edited the West Riding Medical Reports; he also enforced necropsies as a routine and started a laboratory for anatomy, neuropathology, histology, and for animal experimentation. He invited senior students from the Leeds Medical School for demonstrations and tutorials which he often conducted himself.[2]

Undergraduate education

In Britain there was little support for the teaching of psychiatry from the government, universities or medical schools (the last were assemblies of senior doctors in private practice who gave most of their time to earning their living, with less to their hospital and students and even less to research). In the case of psychological medicine, general hospitals would not usually admit psychiatric patients (asylums were geographically separate) and were averse to allowing them as out-patients. When psychiatry emerged as a specialty in the 1870s, its practitioners were kept out of the clinical schools, and only very gradually admitted to hospitals, against the resistance of general physicians and surgeons.

When London University was privately founded in 1826 as a non-sectarian University College, and established a medical faculty, there were at first no clinical facilities. John Conolly, the first Professor of Medicine (1828), was already specialising in mental illness and tried, like some medical professors elsewhere (Pinel in Paris, Griesinger in Germany, later Laycock in Edinburgh), to provide lectures and clinical experience in this field. However, there were no psychiatric patients in Gower Street, and he failed to get his medical students in anywhere else. As he was expected to support his family by London private practice he resigned his chair in 1830.

In 1865 Maudsley persuaded the Convocation of the University of London to resolve that instruction in mental diseases should be required for the final Bachelor of Medicine examination. A number of lectureships were created at various medical schools, usually held by members of the Association. Conolly lectured at Charing Cross Hospital from 1852, Blandford at St George's from 1871, Crichton-Browne at St Mary's from 1881. One lecturer, Edgar Sheppard, of Colney Hatch, even had the title of professor at King's College Hospital. Maudsley, who was professor of forensic medicine at University College Hospital, probably covered mental disorder in his course

---

2   Online archive 8. Sir James Crichton-Browne.

of lectures. These lecturers were outsiders; none of them held appointments as physicians to the hospitals concerned. At Guy's Hospital in 1871 (Sir) George Savage, an old Guy's student and leading London specialist, was appointed as their first lecturer in mental physiology in relation to mental disorder. He was admitted to the hospital staff as a physician 25 years later, but was never allowed to conduct an out-patient clinic, or to have any in-patients in the hospital.

In Edinburgh, however, the development that Morison had instituted was later continued by Laycock (professor of medicine) at the University of Edinburgh and in 1864, at the conclusion of his optional course of lectures, he emphasised the progress made in psychiatry in the previous quarter of a century: 'the visits of a class of students to an asylum are much more beneficial than injurious, if injurious at all; and ... it would greatly conduce to the better knowledge of insanity, and the better treatment of the insane, if the practical study of mental disorders and defects was not limited to the medical profession, but was included in the course of training of other professions.'[3] This was taken up by the Association in their endeavours to train and educate nurses, as described in the previous chapter.

Psychiatrists working in mental hospitals deplored the fact that most of those practising this branch of medicine had had no special instruction for the work they were expected to carry out. They argued that psychiatric patients should be admitted to acute units of general hospitals so that students could become acquainted with the sort of emergency they might encounter in practice. The neuroses at this time were dealt with by general physicians. In 1885, Edward Moore, an Irish psychiatrist, in an address to the MPA dealt with some familiar objections to the teaching of psychological medicine.[4] He considered, for example, the fear that another subject might be piled onto the already lengthy medical curriculum: his rejoinder was 'omit a subject of less importance'. He believed that there was already a change of public opinion which would compel psychiatrists to be better trained in their specialty.

In 1875 and again in 1879 Clouston moved that an approach should be made to the GMC, and accordingly the general secretary, Henry Rayner, wrote to the Council urging that mental diseases should be made a subject of examination for all medical qualifications. The GMC replied that mental disorder was already part of regular courses in medicine, but declined to have it made the subject of a separate examination. In 1885 the GMC added mental disease as a separate item in the curriculum and also ruled that knowledge of all separate items should be tested; this was from then on usually done by means of a single question in the medicine papers.

3   Laycock, T. (1863) The Edinburgh teaching of psychology. *JMS*, **9**, 444.
4   Moore, E. E. (1885) On the necessity of all medical students attending lectures in psychological medicine. *JMS*, **31**, 38.

Postgraduate qualifications

In 1885 the Medico-Psychological Association decided to institute a postgraduate Certificate in Psychological Medicine (CPM). Among the rules for sitting the examination were three months' residence in a mental hospital and attendance at lectures on insanity. Nobody took the examination, so the rules were made still easier. Then 13 people took the examination, and by 1896 about 240 persons held the Certificate. In 1888 it was awarded to a woman for the first time (Jane Waterston, of Cape Town). This was regarded as a precedent for the admission of women to the membership of the Association. The Certificate was never very popular, as it was narrow in scope and depended more on vocational than academic knowledge. Clouston therefore suggested the establishment in Edinburgh of a postgraduate diploma which would deal with the anatomy, physiology and pathology of the brain, psychology, neurology and mental diseases. Diplomas in psychological medicine were instituted by various examining bodies from about 1911 onwards. In 1948 the CPM was finally abolished and replaced by a Diploma in Psychological Medicine. This ran from 1948 to 1959, by which time 29 candidates had passed it. It was not successful and was abolished in its turn.

The Gaskell Prize and bronze medal

After the death of Samuel Gaskell in 1886 his sister, Mrs Holland, acting through his trustees, made over to the MPA a sum sufficient to provide for the annual award of a Gaskell Gold Medal and money prize. At first candidates for the Association entry examination, provided they had qualified medically, were allowed to take an additional 'honours' paper; the prize was awarded on the result of this higher examination. A few examples have survived of the papers set for the entry and 'honours' examinations. (The questions for the 1895 examination are given in online archive 27. Question paper) In later years the 'Gaskell' was kept entirely separate from the MPC and an ad hoc examination of a higher (and continually rising) standard was instituted. The first award, in 1887, went to J. E. D. Mortimer of Portsmouth City Asylum; he left psychiatry not long afterwards, but in the following year the winner was T. B. Hyslop of Bethlem, later well known for his works on psychiatric history and biography, and as a musician.

The MPA Bronze Medal and Prize, instituted in 1882, was awarded for the best dissertation on a clinical or pathological subject related to mental disorder. The first winner of the prize, J. Wigglesworth of Rainhill, made many further contributions to the Journal and was the MPA president in 1902. Another notable winner was George Robertson, of Morningside, Edinburgh, who was awarded the medal and the prize in 1892 and subsequently became professor of psychological medicine at Edinburgh and was president of the MPA in 1922.

A university-linked teaching hospital

In 1908 Henry Maudsley proposed that there should be created a hospital providing early treatment, research and teaching in association with a university. Dr D. G. Thompson (later president of the MPA for the duration of the First World War) seized on this and declared that

'I am absolutely convinced that the success of any scheme of reform in the medical aspect of asylum or rather lunacy work depends entirely upon the provision of definite post-graduate training of our future alienists, and this post-graduate training can only be organised and rendered effective if it is instituted by the universities or other teaching bodies as suggested by Dr Maudsley and a diploma in mental medicine can be granted, without which no one can aspire to lunacy work or appointments.'[5]

The outline of desirable training included one- or two-year study of the anatomy and physiology of the nervous system, neuropathology, experimental psychology normal and morbid (such as that done by Drs Sherrington, Rivers and others), and of course systematic and clinical psychiatry.

'All those subjects could be taught in wards and laboratories of a mental hospital, such as Dr Maudsley proposes in London, and afterwards in similar institutions in the great teaching centres Edinburgh, Dublin etc. ... Dr Maudsley does not write loose English: he must have had some comparative idea in his mind as between what is in vogue in the way of psychiatric instruction at present, and what psychiatric instruction ought to be in his use of the word "good" before the word "instruction."'[6]

Following further debate about this in the MPA, Mercier in 1910 wrote, as president, to all the examining bodies in Great Britain and Ireland (i.e. the universities and colleges):

'It has long been felt by those most intimate with the subject that there is in this country no adequate systematic instruction in psychiatry. The evils of this neglect become year by year more and more manifest. This Association is impressed with the urgent necessity for post-graduate teaching in psychiatry in medical schools; and for the granting of a special diploma to candidates after examination, as has already been done with such conspicuous success in public health and tropical medicine. The position of psychiatry as a branch of medicine is unsatisfactory; it is not properly affiliated to other departments of medicine, to their mutual detriment; and under present conditions cannot make full use of those modern methods of research which have resulted in such advances in general medicine.'[7]

---

5   Thomson, D. G. (1908) The teaching of psychiatry. *JMS*, **54**, 550–555.
6   ibid.
7   Mercier, C. (1910) Postgraduate curriculum in psychological medicine. *JMS*, **56**, 373.

A number of universities responded by authorising courses of instruction and an examination leading to a diploma. Several psychiatrists hoped that the new scheme would keep medical officers' minds keen and on a higher level, raise the ethical standard, dignity and importance of psychiatry. By 1913 a review of the facilities for teaching psychiatry in the various medical schools showed some advance, not so much in regard to the undergraduates as in the provision of courses for those doctors who wished to take the diploma. This consisted mainly of lectures, and postgraduate clinical instruction does not appear to have been available in more than one or two places (Edinburgh, Cambridge). In 1914 a detailed review by Bedford Pierce disclosed a gloomy situation. To summarise, there was little organised teaching, few asylums had laboratories, no scientific career was available in psychiatry, and disparaging comparison was made between arrangements for postgraduate study in this country and those available at Johns Hopkins (Baltimore) under Adolf Meyer and at the Munich University under Kraepelin.

In 1923 the Maudsley Hospital was opened for the purposes that Maudsley had had in mind when he endowed it and courses of instruction, organised by Frederick Mott, were instituted. These were designed to prepare people for a diploma based on intensive courses of lectures and demonstrations lasting six months. Besides members of the hospital staff, the lecturers included prominent teachers of the various subjects, like Bernard Hart, Alfred Tredgold, William Norwood East, Hubert Bond. Doctors flocked to the courses because they were the only comprehensive preparation available for anyone who wanted to take a diploma in psychiatry, although some systematic instruction was also provided in Edinburgh. In spite of the distinguished lecturers, the annual postgraduate courses at the Maudsley were in practice cram courses and did little more than ensure that those who attended them would acquire a good deal of pre-digested information. The diploma course had some obvious defects, not least from the gulf that then existed between the teachers on the course and the examiners for university diplomas (DPMs) or the Conjoint Diploma awarded jointly by the Royal College of Physicians and Royal College of Surgeons. The best commentary on the diploma as it existed in the 1920s and 1930s is contained in the opening paragraph of the Royal College of Physicians Report in 1944:

'The institution of a diploma in psychological medicine in 1910 did much to raise the level of psychiatry in this country. It obliged most of the doctors who work in mental hospitals to acquire a basic knowledge of their subject, and it wiped away the old reproach that there were psychiatrists who had little psychiatry and less psychology. But an advance, however valuable, may fall short of what the times require. Even with the DPM established as the requisite for promotion in the mental hospitals service, there were still many psychiatrists outside the mental hospitals who had not had this basic training; and inside the mental hospitals there were psychiatrists insufficiently equipped by clinical experience and training for work in outpatient departments and child guidance clinics. The causes of this were not simple, but prominent among them must be reckoned the relatively low standard and range of the DPM requirements. A young doctor could obtain the diploma within a year after qualifying if he chose, and could do this without any remarkable abilities or extraordinary application, nor indeed need he have had anything to do as a doctor with the large group of mental disorders called neuroses.'[8]

The most powerful influence in bringing about a direct change in psychiatric education, both for postgraduates and for medical students, was provided in 1944 by the Report of the Interdepartmental Committee on Medical Schools (the Goodenough Committee). Their recommendations in regard to the proper incorporation of psychiatry into the undergraduate curriculum brought long-awaited change, though this took a long time to occur.

Between 1920 and 1970 training in psychoanalysis, analytical psychology and other forms of systematised psychotherapy also developed slowly. In 1935 T. A. Ross devoted the *Morison Lectures*, which he delivered in Edinburgh, to the theme of how the neuroses should be taught to medical students. He hit out against psychoanalysts and psychiatrists with impartial vigour. He took it for granted that physicians in mental hospitals were not likely to be well fitted to run out-patient clinics or to treat in their hospitals people with neurotic disorders. Consequently, he disputed the widespread opinion that general training in psychiatry should be a preliminary to such specialisation as psychotherapy entailed. In his words, '[t]he treatment necessary for the neuroses must always be active. There is an enemy to be routed. The treatment for the psychoses will seldom be active, but will as a rule be mainly on the lines of taking care of and leading the patient gently on.'[9]

The College took up responsibility for postgraduate education in 1972 with a new examination (the Membership of the Royal College of Psychiatrists, MRCPsych) as well as inspection and accreditation of all postgraduate teaching in psychiatry. It was only at this time that the successor to the old Associations became effectively involved in medical education and training.

References and further reading

Crammer, J. (1996) Training and Education in British Psychiatry (1770–1970). In *150 Years of British Psychiatry*, Vol. 1 (The Aftermath) (eds. F. Freeman & G. E. Berrios), pp. 209–242. Athlone Press.

Lewis, A. (1964) Psychiatric Education: Background and History. In *The State of Psychiatry: Essays and Addresses*. Routledge & Kegan Paul. pp. 113–137.

---

8   Royal College of Physicians Committee on Psychological Medicine (1967) Second Interim Report. In *The State of Psychiatry: Essays and Addresses* (ed. A. Lewis). Routledge & Kegan Paul. pp. 119–120.

9   Ross, T. A. (1935) Morison Lectures. *Edinburgh Medical Journal*, **42**, 445.

CHAPTER 13

Journals and other College publications

The idea of establishing a journal was first mentioned at the York Meeting of the Association in 1844 but the decision to do so was postponed to 1852. The first issue of the *Asylum Journal* was published in 1853, later changing its name to the *Journal of Mental Science* and finally becoming the *British Journal of Psychiatry* in 1983. This was an unfortunate decision since 'British' is not 'worldwide' and 'psychiatry' is much narrower a term than 'mental science'. Without this change it might have become the most prestigious psychiatric journal in the world. The *Psychiatric Bulletin*, now a separate publication, evolved from being a section in the Journal under various names, and continues to publish College thinking on mental health policy and to provide a forum for discussion on issues of interest and concern to members. In 1994 *Advances in Psychiatric Treatment* was started to tie in with the College's approach to continuing professional development (CPD), and has flourished ever since. The book programme, originally under the Gaskell imprint, was established in the 1970s, and its development has accelerated since 1986, to over 120 titles in total.

The Journal

The decision to establish a journal and to appoint Dr John Bucknill as editor was taken at the annual meeting of the Association in Oxford in 1852. The Association had been in existence for 11 years, the membership was small and attendance at annual meetings low. The early intention of a three-day annual meeting to include detailed inspection of a mental hospital had been abandoned and in some years no meeting was held. The establishment of the Journal was a bold step, yet one that was justified by events and led, through a series of stages and titles (see Table 13.1), to the *British Journal of Psychiatry*.

The establishment of the Journal was not, however, without its critics. Foremost among these was Dr Forbes Winslow who, five years earlier, had started an independent quarterly *Journal of Psychological Medicine*, published from 1848 to 1860.

Forbes Winslow's objections

The following extract illustrates why Forbes Winslow felt slighted:

Table 13.1. From *Asylum Journal* to the *British Journal of Psychiatry*

Journal	Established (year)	Number of volumes
Asylum Journal	1853	Volume 1, numbers 1–14
Asylum Journal of Mental Science	1855	Volumes 2–4
Journal of Mental Science	1858	Volumes 5–108
British Journal of Psychiatry	1963	Volumes 109–192 (as of January 2008)

'An attempt is now being made to resuscitate a suggestion made last year, at the meeting held at Oxford, in relation to the establishment of a journal in connection with the Association of Medical Officers of Asylums for the Insane. The Editor of this Journal is indebted to the courtesy of a friend for a copy of Dr Bucknill's circular, having reference to this subject. We have a right to ask, why this circular was distributed to other members of the Association, and carefully withheld from ourselves? Again, how was it that the whole plan of the new Journal was conceived, and even its editor selected, before the meeting of the Association last year at Oxford?

We understand that few members of any influence or status in that Association have responded favourably to Dr Bucknill's circular. Many distinguished members have distinctly informed us that they have positively refused to write for it, on the ground that a second psychological journal is not needed. We must confess we do not feel ourselves complimented at the suggestion to establish a periodical of the kind. Our pages have always been open to the communications of the members of the Association, and we have done our utmost to promote its well-being, to advance medico-psychological literature and to support the interest of those connected with the public asylums of this country. Having embarked a capital of some thousand pounds in establishing this journal, and having, since 1848, stood nearly alone in fighting the battle for the British psychologist, it cannot be otherwise than mortifying that those who have never lifted their little finger to assist us, should, in 1853, attempt to injure the property of this journal by starting a rival publication.'[1]

The matter was subsequently resolved amicably and within four years Forbes Winslow had been elected president of the Association.

The *Asylum Journal*

The *Asylum Journal* was published at six-weekly intervals until July 1855. Each issue had 16 pages, the format was 'royal 8vo' and the journal was

---

1   Winslow, F. (1853) *Journal of Psychological Medicine and Mental Pathology*, **6**, 453–455.

printed in two columns with a price of sixpence per copy. The 14 early numbers constitute the first volume. The first issue began with a prospectus by the editor, Dr Bucknill:

'From the time when Pinel obtained the permission of Couthon to try the humane experiment of releasing from fetters some of the insane citisens chained to the dungeon walls of the Bicêtre to the date when Conolly announced that, in the vast Asylum over which he presided, mechanical restraint in the treatment of the insane had been entirely abandoned, and superseded by moral influence, a new school of special medicine has been gradually forming. That period which is marked in the annals of France as the Reign of Terror saw the star of hope arise over the living sepulchre of the lunatic. Pinel vindicated the rights of science against the usurpations of superstition and brutality; and rescued the victims of cerebro-mental disease from the exorcist and the gaoler. But the victory was not gained in one battle; the struggle was carried on with unabating success, until in this country the good work was definitely consummated by the labours of Conolly.

The Physician is now the responsible guardian of the lunatic, and must ever remain so unless by some calamitous reverse the progress of the world in civilisation should be arrested and turned back in the direction of practical barbarism. Since the public in all civilised countries have recognised the fact that Insanity lies strictly within the domain of medical science, new responsibilities and new duties have devolved upon those who have devoted themselves to its investigation and treatment. Many circumstances have tended, not indeed to isolate cerebro-mental disease from the mainland of general pathology; but to render prominent its characteristics and to stamp it as a specialty.

Since in the so-called psychical mode of cure, one personality has to act upon another, and since in this case the vehicle, as it were, in which the medicine is exhibited is the person of the administering physician himself this is the first point to be considered. His circumstances (that is, those of the psychiatric physician) must be such as to allow him to devote himself more or less exclusively to this branch of medicine; that is, to give it the greater portion of his time, which is more necessary in this than in other branches, because the treatment in most instances demands a second education. He must be able by his personal demeanour to obtain influence over the minds of other men, which though in fact an essential part of a physician's mode of cure, is a gift that nature often refuses to the most distinguished men, and yet without which mental diseases, however thoroughly understood, cannot be successfully treated.

The necessity of such exclusive devotion to the study of Insanity, of such a second education, would by itself of necessity constitute diseases of the mind into a strict specialty: and it would be difficult to instance any physician, who has ever become celebrated in the treatment of mental disease, or has written any work of standard authority thereon, who has not previously separated himself from the wide field of general medicine.'[2]

---

2   Bucknill, J. (1853) Prospectus. *Asylum Journal*, **1**, 1–7.

Aims and objectives

The aims and objectives of the *Asylum Journal* were then described in the following terms.

'The aims and objects of the Asylum Journal will be, to afford a medium of communication between men engaged in the construction and management of asylums, in the treatment of the insane, and in all subsidiary occupations; it will therefore embrace topics, not only interesting to medical men, but to visiting asylum architects, and chaplains; nothing will be excluded which is not foreign to the modern system of the care and treatment of the insane. It will be a record of improvements and experiments in psychotherapeutics; whether in medicine, hygiene, diet, employment and recreation; or in the construction, fitting, organisation and management of asylums. It will notice new opinions in psychology of the nervous system, and the neurological observations and discoveries of every kind.

It is hoped that it will afford a means of conveying to Visiting Justices and others in whose hands is vested the ultimate authority in the government of asylums, much valuable information respecting their own duties, which has not hitherto reached them through any other channel. That the governing bodies of lunatic asylums and hospitals are much in need of some instruction respecting the principles on which their duties should be discharged is sufficiently evident, from the imperfect arrangements both of accommodation and management still to be found in many asylums; from the excessive expenditure which has often been permitted in the architectural departments and the contrasting, but not counteracting, parsimony in matters more immediate affecting the welfare of the patients.'[3]

Second issue

The second issue contained a summary of the Lunatic Asylum Act 1853 and a note by John Conolly in reply to German criticism of the non-restraint system. With this the *Asylum Journal* was launched with a discussion of what was a central topic in the specialty of the time. Subsequent issues contained much controversy between the total restraint abolitionists (of whom the editor was one) and the defenders of occasional restraint. There were reviews of asylum reports and correspondence on a variety of subjects. Lawsuits were reported, local scandals explored and there was an impressive body of clinical and pathological contributions.

First year of publication

The establishment of the *Asylum Journal* was discussed at the Association's meeting on 22 June 1854. The editor stated that members should judge for themselves but, from many letters he had received, he himself felt that the first year of publication had been a success.

3   ibid.

133

'If [the editor] were tempted to make the slightest complaint that he had not been well supported, the number of original papers from different members of this Association, which the Journal already contained, would at once refute him. He trusted that Members would continue to supply him with similar communications in increasing numbers, and that they would bear in mind Dr Conolly's remarks when, at the Oxford Meeting, they determined to establish the Journal that their case-books of asylums contained an unworked mine of golden wealth which it was their duty to make productive for the public good.'[4]

Dr Forbes Winslow, the main critic of the establishment of the *Asylum Journal*, was generous in his comments. As things had worked out he did not consider it to be a rival to his own journal and he begged to move that '[t]he best thanks of this Association be given to Dr Bucknill, for the manner in which he has conducted the Asylum Journal.'[5]

Change of title

In 1855 the title of the journal was changed to the *Asylum Journal of Mental Science*, the format was altered and it was published quarterly. In 1858 it became known simply as the *Journal of Mental Science*, a name it retained until 1962. In the 1856 treasurer's report it was pointed out that the annual income of the Association almost exactly met its liabilities, including publication of the quarterly issues of the *Journal* in its improved and more expensive form, and a plea was made to the membership to encourage colleagues to subscribe and submit papers for publication. It was the wish of the 1860 meeting that a paid-for digest of foreign psychological literature should be inserted into the journal each quarter and this was agreed.

Editors

There was a change of editor in 1862. Dr Bucknill had been appointed Chancery Visitor by the Lord Chancellor and, therefore, resigned. A special meeting was held in September that year to elect him an honorary member of the Association. Dr Robertson, the current secretary, was appointed Dr Bucknill's successor as editor and when re-elected the following year, requested that Dr Henry Maudsley be associated with him as joint editor. This was agreed and thus Volume 8 was edited by Dr Robertson and Volume 9 jointly.

The list of 19th-century editors of the *Journal* was impressive and included Henry Maudsley, Lockhart Robertson, Thomas Clouston, Hack Tuke, George H. Savage, Henry Rayner – who were seen as fierce and outspoken. As the first editor, John Bucknill perhaps deserves a special mention as the person who brought the Journal into being and was solely responsible for it for ten years. During this time he wrote about 60 personal contributions, brought

---

4   Transactions (1854) *Asylum Journal*, **1**, 88.
5   ibid.

out several books, collaborated in producing the best-known textbook of psychiatry of the period, *The Manual of Psychological Medicine*, superintended the Devon County Asylum and organised the Devon Volunteers.[6]

Rancorous dispute

At the 1876 annual meeting a dispute over the editorship broke out. It was proposed that the joint editors, Dr Maudsley and Dr Clouston, should be reappointed on the grounds that 'the conducting and editorship of the Journal has given general satisfaction,' and the motion was seconded.[7]

At that point Dr Harrington Tuke intervened and stated that the secretary had received a letter from Dr Bucknill, the first editor, that he thought should be read to the meeting before any decision was taken. The secretary protested that he had considered the letter to be confidential and that he had not, therefore, brought it with him. Dr Tuke then outlined the gist of its contents – that Dr Bucknill was willing to offer himself as editor again in the event of Dr Maudsley's resignation – and asked that this should be placed on record and then read and minuted at a subsequent meeting.

Dr Tuke continued:

'I am not myself personally entirely satisfied with the way the Journal is at present conducted. The great literary abilities of the editors are unquestionable: I think no one could say the Journal could be better edited, or be done with greater pains, and perhaps better success, but there are certain doctrines taught there, certain tenets, which are contrary and repugnant to me, and I may say, some others here. I think it would be an advantage year by year to let them see that the Association is watching their proceedings quite prepared to let other fresh men in, or, at all events, not to submit their judgment entirely to the hands to the editors. I venture to say that the present editor or editors of the Journal in their doctrines do not represent the majority of the Association. I shall end by a motion, and I shall ask for the ballot in this case. I shall move that Dr Bucknill, Dr Clouston and Dr Hack Tuke, if he will allow himself to be nominated, should be the editors of the Journal for the ensuing year. I understand that Dr Maudsley proposes to resign next January, and that will at once raise the question. The result of the ballot will show you how just I am in the observations I have made.'

Dr Tuke may have believed Maudsley to be a cynical free-thinker. His amendment was seconded by Dr Murray Lindsay who felt 'that the Journal has not done for the Association what it might have done, what it ought to have done, and what it was expected to have done.'

This was clearly a very difficult situation. Dr Maudsley, Dr Tuke's main target and also his brother-in-law, was present and it was suggested that he should be asked to clarify his position. It was not widely known that he intended to retire and certainly not as soon as January. Dr Rogers, who had

---

6   Online archive 6. John Bucknill.

7   This and the following quotations in this section are from the account of the Annual Meeting in the *Journal of Mental Science* (1876), **22**, 487–503.

originally proposed the continuation of the present editors, protested that since the resignation had not been on the agenda, it should not be discussed and contended that 'Dr Harrington Tuke's motion has placed this meeting in a most invidious position ... the point I rise to is one of order. Is any member in order in speaking to a motion not before the meeting?'

After some discussion on procedures, Dr Maudsley was asked to speak. He said that it has been well known privately to some members of the Association for some time that he had wanted to retire from the editorship after some 15 or 16 years, although he was not aware of having specified January as the time when he would go – 'the first information that I have had on that subject has been from Dr Harrington Tuke; but probably he knows my mind better than I do myself on that matter.'

This slightly barbed comment lightened the atmosphere with laughter but the meeting remained uncomfortable. Maudsley then claimed that some 'very influential members of the Association' had asked him to continue in post for at least another year while the matter of successors was decided. He was happy to do that, or to resign, whichever the Association decided.

Thomas Clouston (co-editor) and Hack Tuke (proposed as a third editor by his namesake, Harrington Tuke) both declined to accept nomination if Maudsley resigned. It was then proposed that, to get over the difficulty, they might appoint J. Bucknill and Hack Tuke in addition to the current two editors, making a total of four. Henry Maudsley then intervened again to state his view that it would be exceedingly unwise to appoint four editors: 'According to my experience two editors are one too many ... I am willing to continue my services with Dr Clouston for the present, but not with more editors.'

There then followed what can only be described as a rancorous dispute with several members expressing their dismay that Harrington Tuke had put them in such an unpleasant position and he himself persisting in his efforts to force a change of editor. In the end two votes were taken. The first was to choose between two editors or one when 24 of those present voted for two and 13 in favour of one. Despite Harrington Tuke's protestations, the second ballot resulted in a clear majority of 19 (28 for and 9 against) in favour of the original motion that the present editors, H. Maudsley and T. Clouston, be re-elected.

More recent developments

In 1938 a committee of the RMPA decided that the Journal should have an editor-in-chief and two co-editors, and appointed G. W. T. H. Fleming to the former position. Dr Fleming held this post for 23 years, finally standing down because of ill health in 1961. His successor, Dr Eliot Slater, introduced specialist assessment of papers and raised the scientific standard of the Journal.

Subsequent editors, Edward Hare and John Crammer improved the Journal finances, transforming a loss-making operation into one that started to generate income for the College. Hugh Freeman continued this progress, bringing more of the journal administration in house (at this time the printers were contributing greatly to the running of the Journal, and benefiting correspondingly from its income), and launching a series of supplements. Up to this point the technical editing had been carried out on a strictly amateur basis by members of the editorial board; the first professional scientific editor was employed in 1987. Throughout this era and that of Hugh Freeman's successor, Greg Wilkinson, the quality, standing, and international reach of the journal continued to rise. The growth of the internet transformed the world of journal publishing, and the *British Journal of Psychiatry* launched its online edition, hosted at the HighWire Press alongside the *BMJ* and other world-class journals, in 2000. The online version has continued to mature rapidly, and new features and functions are being added up to the present.

Psychiatric Bulletin

The *Psychiatric Bulletin* began as a section of the *Journal of Mental Science* and, like the Journal itself, has undergone a number of changes of name and format over the years. It was for many years a miscellany within the Journal, containing news of MPA meetings, articles on topical matters, reprints of press articles, and obituary notices. Later most of the short commentaries were transferred to a more prominent position under the title *Occasional Notes of the Quarter*. In the course of time *News and Notes*, as it had come to be known, was filled almost entirely with official reports of RMPA meetings, and in 1936 it was decided to issue this section as a separate supplement available only to members.

With the formation of the Royal College of Psychiatrists in 1971, Dr Alexander Walk successfully proposed that there should be a newsletter as an adjunct to the scientific content of the Journal. He then played a major role in nursing the project through its formative stages, both as editor and as a one-man pressure group to persuade Council to give financial support at a time of considerable stringency. His personal authority and profound knowledge of the history of the College was vital during the first ten years of publication.

News and Notes aimed to reflect official College policy as well as providing a forum for individual comment on issues of current interest. In July 1977, the title was changed to *Bulletin of the Royal College of Psychiatrists* and in October 1988 to the *Psychiatric Bulletin*. It is circulated to College members along with the *British Journal of Psychiatry*, and to about 285 subscribers, predominantly in the UK and Ireland. With the gradual expansion in sise from 12 pages per issue initially to 40 A4 pages, the scope of the content has broadened considerably. Regular features are interviews with distinguished colleagues and politicians, a correspondence column, conference reports, historical sketches and obituaries, sensitively edited by Henry Rollin. Satirical humour was found in the early years in the form of the Scribe's column.

As the Bulletin became established, the volume of unsolicited material increased exponentially so that original peer-reviewed papers on clinical innovation and developments, medico-political topics, educational, management and ethical issues now appear on a regular basis. It carries the subtitle the 'Journal of Psychiatric Practice' and this is indicative of its progression from a collection of announcements to a fully fledged journal in its own right.

Various editors have made distinctive contributions to the Bulletin's development. John Crammer, through his own contributions and his meticulous attention to those of others, encouraged economy and clarity in writing. Hugh Freeman expanded its scope and international coverage and he and Brian Barraclough acted as two of the main interviewers. Sidney Bloch initiated the Trainees Forum section and the ethical column and also played a major part in commissioning reports on psychiatry in other countries. For the future, the *Psychiatric Bulletin* is set to continue to publish College thinking on mental health policy affairs and to provide a platform for colleagues to ventilate issues of current interest and concern.

Advances in Psychiatric Treatment

This journal was launched in September 1994 in response to growing concern about continuing professional development. A secondary rather than a primary research journal, it publishes commissioned articles giving concise and clear overviews of carefully chosen subject areas in psychiatry. Originally running to 32 pages and with a few hundred subscribers, *Advances in Psychiatric Treatment* grew steadily and healthily under its launch editor, Andrew Sims, and currently publishes 80-page issues and has nearly 3000 subscribers. Unlike the *British Journal of Psychiatry* and the *Psychiatric Bulletin*, it is not free to members. Several years after its launch, the journal was co-opted into the College's official continuous professional development programme and provided as part of the overall programme fee. Later, when the fee was dropped, the journal became free-standing again. Its aims, as expressed in the original proposal, were to provide a useful educational resource for members and generate income for the College, and it has succeeded well in both of these.

Gaskell Press and RCPsych Publications

Beginning with *Recent Developments in Schizophrenia* (eds. A. Coppen & A. Walk, 1967), through the late 1960s and 1970s the College published an occasional series of 'special publications' of the *British Journal of Psychiatry*. These largely followed the format and style of the Journal, although they were sold separately as books rather than distributed with it. In the late 1970s several titles with a more 'book-like' appearance and approach were published. One of the first of these was the first edition of the *Use of Drugs in*

Psychiatry (1978) written by J. Crammer, B. Barraclough & B. Heine, the 5th edition of which is still in print. When the College first started publishing these books, there was some concern that the content should not be seen as representing formal College policy. This would otherwise be extremely restrictive in terms of the types of books that the College would be able to publish and the approval procedures that would need to be adopted. The imprint 'Gaskell', in honour of Samuel Gaskell, was therefore chosen to indicate a degree of distance between the College and the book list. Publication of new titles was extremely sporadic throughout the following decade, and there was never a large enough list to benefit from a combined marketing campaign. In 2007 the College imprint changed from Gaskell to RCPsych Publications.

The book list dates from 1986, when the *Biology of Depression* (ed J. F. W. Deakin) and *Contemporary Issues in Schizophrenia* (eds. A. Kerr & P. Snaith) were published. Shortly after this date the *British Journal of Psychiatry* acquired a full-time scientific editor, and the infrastructure was in place to quickly develop and produce more titles. During the 1990s the Publications Department (as it became) acquired sales and marketing expertise and staff, and developments in technology (particularly the growth of desktop publishing systems) allowed a greater control over the production processes and costs. The list currently runs to about 120 titles in print, with occasional papers as well as a wide variety of mental health information material.

The College website (www.rcpsych.ac.uk)

The College had been aware of the potential of the web early on, and the first College pages (hand coded, and listing basic bibliographic information about the journals) went online in March 1996. These were added to rapidly, and staff were allocated to work on the site part time. A fully redesigned site covering most of the College's functions was launched in November 1998. In June 2000 a full-time administrator was appointed, and further complete redesigns were launched in February 2001 and June 2004.

The Association and later the College have been involved in publishing a journal since 1853 – without this it is doubtful whether the original Association could have survived. With the inception of the College in 1972 this has become much more professional. Further journals and much other publishing (in the Gaskell Press and RCPsych Publications) have been undertaken. The College can be thus seen to be carrying out one of the objects and purposes in its Charter – publishing the results of study and research into the understanding and treatment of mental disorder in all its forms and aspects.

CHAPTER 14

The library and information service

Origins

In January 1863 the Association addressed the question of their having their own library and the following note was published in the *Journal*:

'The President and Committee desire to bring before the Association the question of gathering a small library composed of the English and Foreign Journals of Insanity, of asylum reports and similar papers, to which hereafter, by purchase or donation, the standard works in psychology might be added.

Even in London there exists no complete series of these journals and reports, the best collection being that in the College of Surgeons' library. It is self-evident that a complete series of these papers ought to be in the possession of the Association. The same observation applies to the several reports of the Commissioners in Lunacy in England, Scotland, and Ireland.

The editor is endeavouring to arrange a complete series of exchanges with all the journals on insanity published in Europe and America. Again, if the superintendent of each asylum would send a complete set of the published reports and rules of his asylum, a nucleus for the collection would soon be formed. A similar success might, it is hoped, attend the application by this Association to the Commissioners in Lunacy for a copy of their reports. The several parliamentary returns might also readily be obtained, and it is believed that authors (members of the Association and others) would from time to time add copies of their published works to the collection. The Honorary Secretary has placed a room in 37 Albemarle Street at the free disposal of the Association for the safe custody of such a library – a room which will, at all times, be open to the members of the Association who may wish to consult their books. The President and Committee trust, therefore, that this appeal may not be made in vain. They undertake that the reports thus sent shall be bound in their series of years, marked with the name of the Association, and carefully preserved with all other books and documents, which may from time to time be added by gift or otherwise to the library.

The receipt of any reports or books thus presented will be duly acknowledged in the Journal. Dr Erlenmeyer, editor of the Archiv der Deutschen Gesellshaft für Psychiatrie, offers a copy of a large work on 'Asylum Construction' which he has in the press for this proposed library, and there exists both in Germany and France a great willingness on the part of alienist physicians to bring their writings under the notice of their English brethren, so that the editor feels confident that this appeal would be liberally responded to from abroad.'1

The first formal suggestion that the MPA should have its own library was made in 1864 when the then President, Henry Monro, recommended that the MPA should have a London headquarters and a library. There is no record of any action taken on this suggestion and the next recommendation made about two years later that founding a library would be an appropriate use for the MPA's surplus funds did not lead to any action. In 1895 the MPA moved into a room belonging to the Medical Society of London at 11 Chandos Street and the Society's librarian agreed to take over responsibility for the day-to-day running of an MPA library. Following the death of Daniel Hack Tuke in 1895 his widow had presented the MPA with a large amount of books that had been in his possession.[2] In the mid-1890s the Association developed its library. At that time, membership stood at just over 400 and members came from psychiatric institutions throughout the British Isles. Although there is no record of the titles of the books that made up the bequest, judging by those that have remained in the College library, the collection consisted predominantly of contemporary handbooks, monographs and textbooks almost exclusively on psychological medicine; the bequest, apparently, did not include valuable antiquarian works. A Library Committee was established at the Council meeting in July 1895, consisting of H. Rayner, H. J. MacEvoy and the MPA general secretary, Fletcher Beach. Dr Rayner, who had been the MPA president in 1884, was an extremely active and dedicated member of the Committee who contributed to the development of the library until he resigned from the Committee in 1925. That was anything but easy, however – at one point, when he asked the Council for £15 for book repair and cataloguing, he was told he could have only £10 to go on with.

Initially, the Hack Tuke donation proved to be something of a problem to the newly founded Committee, which, in its report to Council in November 1895, described the books as being in 'a state of confusion and disorder and incompleteness'.[3] They lost no time in setting to work on sorting the books and by February 1896 were able to report to Council that 'about 700 volumes were worthy of retention in the library although 350 of these required repair'.[4] The Committee also considered the best means of making the collection of use to the membership and recommended that it could 'only be of use to so scattered a body by being made circulating.' Three months later H. Rayner reported that the books had been catalogued and the typewritten cards had been arranged in an oak tray, adding that the cost of this work, including the tray, was £9.13.6. The librarian to the Medical

1   Proposed library of the Association (1862) *JMS*, **8**, 613.
2   Online archive 7. Daniel Hack Tuke.
3   *Council Minutes* (1895) College archives.
4   *Council Minutes* (1896) College archives.

Society of London had agreed to take on the administrative duties connected with the Association's book collection for an annual fee of £10. At the annual meeting in 1896 Dr Rayner was able to report that all the gifts from Mrs Tuke had been catalogued and arranged in one of the MPA's rooms – the first reference to library accommodation. At this meeting Dr Rayner also acknowledged Dr F. Hay of Perth who made a unique contribution to the collection by designing an unusual commemorative bookplate – it featured a feather motif on a bronze background.

Financial matters were the main feature of Library Committee reports of the following years with requests for small but increasing sums of money to cover administration and accommodation rather than the purchase of books. In 1897 the Hack Tuke Memorial Committee made its approval apparent by agreeing to 'hand over to the MPA the sum of £350 to be vested in trustees, the annual income derived therefrom to be expended in maintaining and increasing the library, of which Dr. Hack Tuke's gift to the Association has proved such a valuable nucleus'.[5] This capital was later invested in New Zealand Stock, maturing in 1940, and was probably reinvested in war bonds. By the turn of the century the library was well established. Other donations of books were received, with those of past presidents, Drs C. Lockhart Robertson and J.C. Bucknill, of particular note. In November 1899 Dr Fletcher Beach, secretary of the Library Committee, informed the Council that a catalogue of books held in the library had been printed and issued to all members. The aim of the Committee that all members should have access to the library was thus achieved.

The librarian

The first reference to the office of librarian can be found in the minutes of the Council meeting of May 1902. The Library Committee recommended that an honorary librarian should be appointed, to 'manage the library in respect to binding, cataloguing and the recommendation of new books for purchase, subject to the approval of the library committee'.[6] However, once again no action was taken, and although the minutes of the 1904 annual meeting record the appointment of Robert Cole as honorary librarian in place of Seymour Tuke, there is no reference to Tuke's own appointment. Cole himself does not seem to have developed a role as the MPA's librarian, for the bye-laws were not altered to include him among the officers and in the list of members of the Library Committee he appears as the secretary or as an ordinary member. Despite this, in 1904 the library, with about 1000 books, was described as one of the most useful parts of the MPA and members were urged to meet the appeals of the Committee for more books in 'an intelligent and liberal spirit.' Until the mid-1920s

5   Hack Tuke Memorial (1897) *JMS*, **43**, 869.
6   *Council Minutes* (1902) College archives.

Library Committee reports as well as record details of book purchase and circulation, accommodation, storage and finance were presented to Council and annual meetings by the secretary of the Committee.

The RMPA library

At the May 1927 Council meeting the president, J. R. Lord, proposed that the bye-laws should be altered to allow the appointment of an honorary librarian. J. R. Whitwell was appointed as acting honorary librarian until the necessary alterations could be made and he was confirmed as the RMPA's first honorary librarian at the November 1928 council meeting, a decision that was loudly applauded; he remained librarian till 1944. Whitwell's successor was only librarian for two years: Alexander Walk replaced him in 1946, remaining in post until 1972.

The College's library ...

With the inception of the College in 1972 Dr Dennis Leigh was elected librarian. When the College moved to Belgrave Square the books were transferred to the basement, where they remained unpacked for some years. The library was developed with shelving for books on the second floor. This required major repairs to the building as steel beams were needed to support the weight of the upper floors. In March 1973 Dennis Leigh reviewed the library's problems in *News and Notes* and Helen Marshall, the librarian at the Institute of Psychiatry, made a similar report. They received what could be described as a haphazard collection of books, and recommended finding what the membership required from their library. Leigh noted that other medical college libraries were basically reference libraries functioning mainly bibliographically providing reference and photostatic facilities to their members. He considered what should be done with the three main types of the library's contents, the books, journals and its historical collection. The library had no budget, no staff and no defined role. There was a need for a professionally qualified librarian on the staff.[7]

... and information service

Despite these early and sensible recommendations it took a long time for the library that passed from the RMPA to the College to develop into the current Library and Information Service. The College's second librarian (the distinguished psychiatric historian Dr Henry Rollin) oversaw the transferring of the remains of the library into its new headquarters on the second floor of Belgrave Square. He was also responsible for obtaining the funds from

---

7   Leigh, D. (1973) The College library. *News and Notes*, March, 1–5.

Council to appoint the first (initially part-time) professional librarian. H. Rollin was followed by another distinguished historian, German Berrios, in the post of honorary librarian. Dr Berrios was anxious to develop the service further with an information service, archive and museum. The first archivist to the College had been appointed on a part-time basis and Dr Berrios with the archivist introduced computers in many of the College's activities as well as completing the cataloguing of the collection. He was succeeded as honorary librarian by Dr Ian Pullen and it was during his tenure of office that the library was extensively modified thanks to a generous gift in memory of the late Dr Josephine Lomax-Simpson (FRCPsych). This included removing out-of-date books and shelving in favour of computer-based working space. Ian Pullen was succeeded in this post by David Tait, who served from 2001 to 2006. His contributions included the transition from a largely paper-based library to an electronic library and information service, the establishment of the College records management system and the launch of a programme to repair and refurbish the College's antiquarian book collection. This is the College's single greatest financial asset, but more important is its intellectual value as a priceless and unique psychiatric, medical and library archive.

It is appropriate to conclude by illustrating how the library matches the three objectives and purposes set out in the College Charter. The first is to promote the science and practice of psychiatry and it is our service to the membership, for instance literature search, article retrieval, access to College documents and policies, etc., which meets this aim. The second is public education and it is the public, primarily users and carers, who are the single biggest user group of the information service. The third is that of promoting study and research and the College Research and Training Unit is also a major user of the service. It is therefore pleasing that the plans outlined by Dennis Leigh in the early days of the College have been fully realised.

CHAPTER 15

Premises

When Samuel Hitch and his five colleagues agreed to form the Association of Medical Officers of Asylums and Hospitals for the Insane in 1841 they did not know that it would grow into an organisation needing its own headquarters. A permanent home is first mentioned in the minutes of the 1864 annual meeting when the president, Dr Munro, suggested that 'If we could get thus into bricks and mortar, and have a more solid existence than at present, that would help to establish us very much.'[1] The meeting decided against this on the grounds that it would make the Association strictly metropolitan. The question was discussed at intervals until 1893 when the MPA began to lease space from the Medical Society of London. The Association and later College were housed for over 80 years in Number 11 Chandos Street (now called Lettsom House), apart from a short sojourn with the British Medical Association (BMA) from 1926 to 1932. The College was also briefly housed in Chandos House (1971–1974). It then moved to its present headquarters in Belgrave Square.

Chandos Street

Robert de Chandois is supposed to have 'come over with William the Conqueror', and several centuries later a daughter of a Herefordshire branch of his family married one Giles Brugges or Brydges. In the 1500s their descendant, Sir John, was made Lord Chandos. In 1719, the 8th Lord Chandos, James Brydges, amassed a huge fortune through holding the post of paymaster to the armed forces under Marlborough, and for this and his services to his political party he was made Duke of Chandos. When the Cavendish Square estate was laid out the 'Grand Duke', as he was already being called, was to occupy the finest position, for a whole block on the north side of the square was to be taken up by a magnificent mansion, with a spacious forecourt and a formal garden at the rear. The streets on either side, running northwards from the square, were to be named 'Chandos Street' and 'Harley Street' (the names were the reverse of what they are now). If this original plan had been adhered to, the site for No. 11 would have been covered by the garden and one of the wings of

---

1   Annual Meeting (1864) *JMS*, **10**, 453.

the Duke's mansion. But the crash of the South Sea Bubble called a halt to development; the mansion never came into being and the two side streets remained for years in a truncated state. Harley Street and Chandos Street changed names because under the revised plan the western street was to be the more important and would bear the name of the estate owner. The new Chandos Street, therefore, became what it is now, a short connecting street ending in a right-angled turn. By 1769 the third Duke was sufficiently prosperous to be able to plan a new town house in the street named after his grandfather. Thus the present Chandos House arose, the work for the most part of Robert Adam.[2]

Lettsom House

About the same time as Chandos House was being built in 1773, the Medical Society of London was funded. The Society's original home was in Bolt Court in the City, but in 1872 it moved to Chandos Street. No. 11, named Lettsom House after the Society's founder, Dr John C. Lettsom, had a Regency appearance and the lettering on the facade suggested that it was purpose-built; but in fact it was bought (with No. 12) by the Society from the Earl of Gainsborough, whose town house it had been. It was completely remodelled to provide meeting rooms and library. The earliest record of a meeting of the MPA at No. 11 can be found in the Journal for October 1886, but at first this was the venue only for London annual meetings, which had previously been held at the Royal College of Physicians. Quarterly meetings continued to be held for the most part at Bethlem. The MPA had at that time no permanent home, but the need for at least a pied à terre in London was strongly felt, and in 1893 it signed an agreement with the Medical Society. The Society, in return for a small rental, granted the following privileges:

- the use of a bookcase to house the embryo library (much augmented a few years later by Hack Tuke's bequest);
- the use of rooms for meetings and committees;
- permission for the general secretary to use the Society's library on occasion for dealing with MPA correspondence;
- permission to use Number 11 as the MPA's official address.

Thereafter, meetings at No. 11 were described in the minutes as having taken place in 'the rooms of the Association'.

The BMA house

The arrangement with the medical Society of London continued until 1926 when the MPA received the Royal Charter. The opening of the new

2   Walk, A. A. (1974) Farewell to Chandos Street. *News and Notes*, 2–4.

BMA house in Tavistock Square appeared to offer an opportunity for better accommodation and so the RMPA moved there in 1926 and remained till 1932. The annual meeting in 1926 was held in the BMA's great hall, and quarterly meetings in their Council Chamber. It was hoped that before long the MPA would have at least one room of its own in the building. These hopes were thwarted, and in 1932 the RMPA returned to 11 Chandos Street. It rented a small office on the ground floor with another room for an office for the first paid part-time secretary.

Back to Lettsom House

After the First World War, there was a good deal of expansion and rearrangement. First, a larger office and a further room for the RMPA library were secured. Later, this room was given up and the library occupied two small rooms adjoining the main office. By 1963 the staff had increased to three, all working in one small office; the Journal was no longer being run from the editor's own hospital; and the membership had more than doubled and was continuing to increase. A series of agreements for extra rooms, preserved in the College archives, show how over the years the work of the RMPA, and its staff, had expanded.

In the early 1960s a move to the Royal College of Physicians' new building in Regent's Park was considered, but instead the RMPA moved from Lettsom House to the Royal Society of Medicine's Chandos House.

Chandos House

Chandos House is one of the few Adam houses still remaining in London. It was built by the brothers Robert and James Adam in 1769 and 1770 for the 3rd Duke of Chandos. The second and third floors of the house were used as offices and the RMPA and later the Royal College of Psychiatrists occupied five large rooms on the second floor from 1965 until 1975. The College's library was used also for Council and committee meetings. With its white and gold wallpaper and semi-circular window with long blue velvet curtains, it retained some of the elegance of the rest of the house, but the other rooms, though they had beautifully moulded plaster ceilings and fireplaces and panelled walls, had lost much of their graciousness through being put to modern uses. Eventually, they became very overcrowded with people, office furniture and equipment, and stationery stocks; the College had far outgrown its accommodation. Fortunately, just when expansion was becoming an urgent matter, the College was able to add three small rooms on the third floor to its premises. These rooms were occupied by the editorial office of the *British Journal of Psychiatry* and the newly formed Examinations Department.

Belgrave Square

The creation in the 1820s of the aristocratic district that came to be known as Belgravia is often attributed solely to the enterprise of the builder and developer Thomas Cubitt, but it appears that the development had been envisaged well before then by the landowners, the Earls Grosvenor (afterwards Marquesses and Dukes of Westminster). The planning of the streets and squares was the work of the architects James Wyatt and Thomas Cundy, and the actual building was carried out by more than one firm: Cubitt, Seth Smith, and for most of Belgrave Square itself by the brothers Haldimand. By the time work was started, London had already extended further west – in a ribbon along Knightsbridge, down Sloane Street and into Hans Town to the South of Brompton Road, so that the site of the future Belgravia was an undeveloped island, the reason being the damp marshy character of the clay soil. There had been a brick kiln near this spot, and the developers used up the whole of the clay stratum to make the bricks they needed, and afterwards they raised the level of the ground by spreading gravelly soil excavated in the construction of St Katharine's Dock in the East End of London, of which one of the Haldimands was a director. The rise from Belgrave Square to Hyde Park Corner is still noticeable to this day.

'Belgrave' itself has an unusual derivation. There is a village of Belgrave in Leicestershire – now a suburb of Leicester and its town hall is a museum; and there is also a hamlet of Belgrave on the Eaton Hall estate. It appears that the original name of the village was 'Merdegrave', signifying 'a grove inhabited by pine-martens', but the occupying Normans thought the first part of the word improper, and so it was euphemised by removing the offensive prefix and substituting the more acceptable 'Bel'. The square deserves the 'bel' prefix, for it is one of the grandest in London. The houses on each side are a single architectural composition, and the style and materials are those made famous earlier in the Regency period by John Nash – a monumental mansion in the centre and wings with a plainer terrace between.[3]

The architect was George Basevi, whose best-known work is probably the Fitzwilliam Museum in Cambridge. He might have gone on to greater things, but was accidentally killed at a comparatively early age. Number 17 is near the centre of the west side. Its previous occupants were slightly less aristocratic than those of some of the other houses. In the mid-19th century it was inhabited by a Member of Parliament, Sir Robert Howard; next by successive members of the Ralli family, for many years by Penteli Ralli, also an MP; during this time Lord Kitchener is stated to have made the house his 'social headquarters'. Next came another MP, A.R. Marriott, and the last private resident was Lady (Leontine) Sassoon, the mother of Sir

---

3   Walk, A. A. (1975) Arrival in Belgrave Square. *News and Notes*, 3–5.

Victor Sassoon. After the Second World War it housed part of the Ministry of Education, and its last owner before the College was the Institute of Metals.[4]

17 Belgrave Square

In 1973 the College's lease of the Royal Society of Medicine's Chandos House was due to expire and could not be extended for more than a few months. There had also been an increase in administrative staff and it was decided to try to find permanent headquarters. Various options were suggested including a move to a property adjoining the Royal College of Physicians, moving outside London, building on a new site in London, and renting or buying within London. A number of properties were considered: St Peter's Hospital in Henrietta Street – 'an attractive brick building'; Queen Mary's Maternity Home, Hampstead – 'solidly built in Neo-Georgian style'; the Moorfields Hospital Highgate Annexe – 'a very respectable residential area'; and the Royal Victoria Patriotic Asylum in Wandsworth – 'originally built to house 300 orphaned daughters of the brave Crimea dead.'[5] Finally a lease was bought on 17 Belgrave Square.

A small Appeals and Buildings Committee was involved in the search in 1973. One of the members (Dr Henry Rollin) knew Edward Sieff of Marks and Spencer and visited him, explaining the new College's problem. The Committee were invited to the headquarters, where the president made a forceful presentation of their need. The Marks and Spencer Foundation responded very positively by promising £100 000, but with the proviso it would have to be used within six months or the offer would be withdrawn. This concentrated the minds of the Committee and an intensive search disclosed that 17 Belgrave Square was on the market, although the College was some £700 000 short of the purchase price. The Appeals Committee, who had to decide, acted with speed and rapidly completed the purchase. Sir Paul Mallinson, a member of the Committee was unhappy about the sise of the debt to be incurred and resigned, doubting it was wise to be so heavily bound. This necessitated a large loan, guaranteed by the College's sponsors Lord Goodman and Lord Rayne. However, the property market at the time was dominated by a large group of avid, ruthless, picaresque characters and the Crown Commissioners and the Church Commissioners were not helpful. (Sir Keith Joseph, however, telephoned Martin Roth on each occasion the Department of Health vacated a building.) This left the College with a substantial debt to repay, with high interest rates. The treasurer seemed at times on the verge of anxiety neurosis. But with the help of some foundations and benefactors the debt was cleared within three

---

4   Williams, M. H. (2000) Belgrave Square in the 20th century – the first fifty years. *Psychiatric Bulletin*, **24**, 34–35.

5   Harcourt Williams, M. (1999) The search for accommodation. *Psychiatric Bulletin*, **23**, 761.

years. The College had acquired a splendid house in a Regency terrace build in 1805 which became its permanent home. The Committee had struck the right balance in acquiring their prestigious headquarters – Martin Roth had made the acquiring of suitable premises a major part of the first years of his presidency. In August 1974 he wrote in *News and Notes* to the membership:

'The College acquired 17 Belgrave Square as its new home and headquarters. After many set-backs and disappointments we have achieved what appeared, at some stages of our quest in these last three years, an unattainable objective. It would not have been possible without generous and unfailing help from our sponsors. And it is difficult to express in words the gratitude which we owe to Lord Goodman, their Chairman, who has managed in an exceedingly busy life to find time and energy to devote to our cause. I know that his efforts have sprung in considerable measure from deep conviction about the importance of psychiatry in the contemporary world.'[6]

When the College acquired 17 Belgrave Square there was much work to be done before they moved there and it became clear that there were opportunities for extending the building. This happened in 1987 at the back and a fourth floor was built to provide additional office space for the new Research Unit and the expanding Examinations and Publishing Departments. In 1997 an extensive refurbishment of the formal rooms started with the aim of meeting both the College's practical needs and enhancing the period detail of its property. The increase in College activities had also led to the Research Unit with its staff of 40 moving to separate premises in Aldgate (following sojourns in Grosvenor Crescent and Victoria Street).

---

6   Roth, M. (1974) Letter from the President. *News and Notes*, 1–4.

Epilogue

The asylum tradition endeavoured to carry out humane treatment for an outcast group – in the 19th century the paragon of such an attitude was Lord Shaftesbury. In the 20th century the most important advances in psychiatry in the UK were made by rational psychiatrists at the hospital that bears Maudsley's name. The 21st century has started with the National Health Service undergoing ever more rapid reorganisations and pressures to reach targets. Having spent some time reviewing the psychiatry of the past two centuries, are there any indications of what the future may hold?

The founders of the Association in 1841 expected that establishing asylums with a new approach to the treatment of the mentally ill would lead to cures, but this did not occur. It is as difficult today as it was for them to forecast future developments. Few of the advances of the past 200 years were foreseen, whether it was the use of malaria and then penicillin to treat cerebral syphilis, the accidental discoveries of drugs that could modify some of the more disabling symptoms of severe forms of mental illness, or the development of measures to evaluate psychotherapeutic and other treatments.

It is reasonable to expect that just as general paralysis of the insane (GPI) has become a rarity, other forms of mental illness that are expressions of cerebral disease will similarly fade away, with relevant advances in therapeutics. We can expect to see further advances in our understanding of the aetiology and pathogenesis of mental disorders. But recent history would suggest that our progress in understanding fundamental psychological processes such as memory, speech and perception will increase only slowly.

In the 1950s psychiatry acquired a series of effective therapies that were all chance discoveries. The therapeutic effects of phenothiazines, tricyclic antidepressants, monoamine oxidase inhibitors and lithium were all discovered fortuitously within a few years of one another by researchers who were looking for something quite different, and our understanding of how these drugs work remains incomplete. We may, of course, acquire other effective and novel therapies in equally fortuitous ways in the future. Hopefully we will eventually acquire potent new therapies, not by luck, but by a rational process of development based on a better understanding of aetiology. The cholinesterase inhibitors currently used for the treatment of Alzheimer's disease may be the harbingers of such developments. Although these appear to be only modestly and temporarily effective, Alzheimer's disease seems closer to yielding some of its secrets than other major psychiatric disorders. Drug companies continue to develop amyloid protease inhibitors or amyloid precursor protein antagonists, and it is possible that a means will be found to prevent or delay the deposition of amyloid. If this happens, with a prevention of the development of the symptoms of this disease, the consequences for the image of the psychiatry of old age – and consequently the status of the psychiatric profession and the future of the College itself – should be as profound as those for patients, their families and the nursing home industry.

Therapeutic advances in the future will not all be pharmacological. In the past few years there has been the development, mainly by clinical psychologists, of more effective psychological therapies for the treatment of anxiety states, for drug-resistant hallucinations and delusions and, perhaps, for reducing the risk of relapse in bipolar disorder. Other effective psychological and social therapies will presumably continue to be developed and deployed. Perhaps psychotherapy will move towards attainment of its aims – a solid theoretical foundation, and communicable methods and techniques that have a well-documented efficacy, well-understood indications for use, and practical applicability to the majority of those who need them.

Will psychiatrists extend or narrow their scope in dealing with social deviation? If the course of events in the last half-century is a guide, they will be asked more and more to deal with criminals, turbulent and disturbed adolescents, and other people who offend against the social canons. There will no doubt be continuing efforts to combat the fear and misunderstanding that colour people's notions of mental illness. I would like to be able to hope that there will be an increasing recognition, by the general public, politicians and the media, of the high prevalence and disabling consequences of mental illness. The ground has been laid by epidemiological research and it will also be brought about by personal experience. If there is a reduction in the stigma associated with mental health problems, and I cannot be hopeful about this, it might eventually result in an increasing willingness, by politicians and the general public, to devote a higher proportion of healthcare spending to the treatment of psychiatric disorders.

Meanwhile, the effects on the College of current trends – such as the increasingly 'biological' nature of psychiatric research, the growing influence of service user-led initiatives, and the proliferation of 'clinical guidelines' – will be for my successor to relate.

The history of the College could not include any thoughts about the future. Similarly, although psychiatrists differ from other doctors, this would be inappropriate in this book. I have therefore provided an online archive which covers both topics.[1]

---

1   Online archive 39. Some personal reflections.

Index

Compiled by Caroline Sheard